How Connie Got Her Rack Back

CONSTANCE BRAMER

Best Wishes
Constance Bramer

D1157466

Back cover photos by Quinton Mulvey

Published by:

FriesenPress
Suite 300 – 852 Fort Street
Victoria, BC, Canada V8W 1H8

www.friesenpress.com

Distributed to the trade by The Ingram Book Company

Dedication

Dear Mom,

I miss you every day that I am able to take a breath. I think often of the life lessons you have taught me: to always be giving, to always be forgiving, and to leave people better for having known me. I hope that I am living up to the example you have set. Every time I smell a flower when none are near, I know it is you. I wrote this book for the both of us.

All my love,

Connie

Dear Dad,

Thank you for always supporting me, teaching me to always do the right thing and loving me through all of it. You are my hero.

Love,

Connie

To my beautiful children Alyssa and Alex,

Thank you for being the most amazing people I know. Remember to always look forward, your face into the sun, letting the light inside you shine through. You are the love and light in my life that guides me. I love you both so very much.

Love,

Mom

Many thanks for the love and support of my friends and family, and a special thanks to *CaringBridge* for providing me with a platform to write my story.

Chapter 1
The News

*I*t's funny how you can be bee-bopping along in your life like a frenzied hamster on a wheel, when all of the sudden, your stupid foot catches on the wheel and you fly off smacking face first into the side of the damn hamster cage. The day I hit the cage face first (and subsequently had bar marks on my face for months) started out like any other day. Seriously, I should have known.

I wake up late (of course) screaming "Get up, get up!" to my kids so they can eat their breakfasts and I won't have to do the dreaded "mom in pajamas signing me into school" bit. They will get on that bus if it KILLS me. I hear the bus coming around the corner, my son the lolly-gagger, taking his sweet time putting on his sneakers. Good grief! Do these kids have a "slow-mo" button? On the bus they go. Some days, the best sight in the world is the tail lights of a yellow school bus—with your kids on it, of course. I know I must sound like a horrible mother for saying so, but hey, it's reality. That and a cosmopolitan can cure almost anything!

So I head to my doctor's office for the much dreaded follow-up mammogram—the one where they find one thousand ways to squeeze your tit like a pancake. I'm an old hat at this. I mean, how many times have I done it? A bunch. You put the ugly gown on with the tie in the FRONT, the x-ray tech holds your breast like a lump of clay and places it on the cold, hard x-ray machine. So pleasant.

Most people need a Xanax to relax. Me, I need a good cup of coffee. I sit on the chair sipping my coffee in my fabulous gown, and read all of the breast cancer statistics posters on the wall. Nothing like some thought-provoking literature to make you even more stressed out while you wait! I sit there thinking of my mother, as I do so often. Here in spirit, I say to her, "Mom, it's not my time for this yet." She knows what I'm talking about, wherever she is. This was her battle too. A valiant effort in her fight, but lost nonetheless.

After I receive a few "pancake shots", the x-ray tech comes back and informs me that the doctor wants more images and she needs to get more film. God, why does this always have to take so long? I have so much to do…the hamster wheel is beckoning. Finally, my photo-op is over. No glamour shots, just malleable films of flecks on a lighted board. The radiologist comes in and tells me that she would like to perform an ultrasound on a couple of spots. No biggie, I've had this done before too.

The ultrasound tech is the human version of Cindy Brady's Chatty Cathy doll. All I'm thinking is get this damn thing over with so I can get back to work and get on with my day! It's amazing to me how we as women have (almost) no modesty after we have birthed children. Gown goes off, boobs exposed, on with the ultrasound.

The goop goes on. Don't they ever warm this stuff up? Chatty Cathy is quiet, so I look up and see that her face is set into a stern expression. What is this about, I wonder. Chatty Cathy is quiet. Chatty Cathy's are not supposed to be quiet. She excuses herself and comes back in with her grim-looking posse.

The radiologist introduces herself, takes the magic wand from Chatty Cathy and runs the lube all over my chest looking for something. The concentration on her face is exhausting me as I watch her. She finally looks up after what seemed like an eight-hour shift, points to a spot and says, "I'm sorry to tell you this, but I believe this is malignant. You will have to have a biopsy to confirm, but I am 99 percent sure this is malignant."

SHUT UP! Why is Chatty Cathy saying "I'm so sorry" with tears in her eyes? Tell me this is some sick joke and Alan Funt is hiding in the corner after I've had my chest exposed to all of American television! Well, Alan's dead, so this is pretty much happening.

Apparently, doctors don't have a great response to, "You're shitting me!" other than to say "I'm sorry" over and over. My first thought is, THIS is my moment? No fanfare, just a room they usher me into akin to a smelly high school classroom with a table, a chair, a box of Kleenex and a phone.

"Can we call anyone for you?"

OH MY GOD! What now? And to think, I was stressed about my kids getting on the bus this morning.

I'd had thoughts of this moment just over a year ago, when I was miserable in my marriage to Dr. Jekyll and Mr. Hyde. I was reaching for a glass out of my cabinet and had an epiphany. I was about to turn 38. I said to myself, "If I live to be the same age as my mother, I have 15 more years left. Do I want to live them like this? HELL NO!" So I got my ducks in a row and got out of Crazyville.

So there I sit, diagnosed with the very illness that prompted me to move on with my life. The irony! I cry, not out of sadness, but more out of disbelief. I call my boyfriend, who is off in a tropical locale "finding himself" for a month. Yeah, that's another version of Crazyville I'll have to fill you in on. I hardly remember the conversation. All I remember thinking was, "Please come home and help me through this."

I don't really want to, but I call my Dad to tell him. I know he will be heartbroken and the floodgates to the past will open up and be unbearably painful. And so I do. While dialing the phone, I think of the car ride during my mother's funeral procession, when the driver said to my father, "Well it's over now," and my father responded, "No, I have my daughter to worry about." So that dreaded day had come to fruition. I remember the heaviness in my father's voice as he said, "I'm sorry."

"I'm so sorry." I know, what else can you say to someone who's just been diagnosed with cancer? "Well, you've made it this far, so I'm sure you'll live." I know that saying "I'm sorry" is a heartfelt sentiment, but it feels empty nonetheless.

No one knows the right thing to say. There is no right thing to say. It just is. It SUCKS, but it is. It's the culmination of every shitty moment you've ever endured in your life all rolled into one.

I walk out to my car in a trance with a feeling of heaviness, yet hollowness at the same time. Like all of the oxygen inside my lungs is being squeezed out of me by a python. The same terrifying feeling I had in college when my boyfriend asked me to hold his snake (no, not THAT one) and it wrapped around me in a vice grip that took two of his friends to help unravel. There was nothing to unravel with this news. Only me.

The whole ride home, I blindly stared ahead. I have no idea how I even got home. I kept saying to myself, "Hi, I'm Connie and I have cancer." Like I was at an AA meeting(not that I've been, although I am probably a few beverages away from a meeting). Cancer, cancer. What the hell?! I feel fine. I look fine. OK, I could look better, but couldn't we all? What woman doesn't want to look a little like Cindy Crawford? As I grapple with all of these thoughts running through my mind, I wonder, "Will I get NEW boobs? New and IMPROVED?" Maybe even a bionic rack.

Then I think of my kids. Oh my god, I can't die! They need me! They can't spend the rest of their lives with Dr. Jekyll or Mr. Hyde as their only parent! I HAVE to live through this, because dying and leaving my kids to be raised in Crazyville is NOT an option! My adrenaline kicks in and I think. I'm back on the hamster wheel. What is the game plan? There must be a game plan. I think back to what the doctor said. Something about having a biopsy. It's scheduled for Friday, two days away. I can live with a little uncertainty for two days, right? She said she's only 99 percent sure it's cancer.

Maybe I can rewind the clock an hour. Just an hour. In that hour's time, my life had turned upside down. If ONLY I could undo this last hour. I am in desperate need of a do-over. I think back to my early 20's when I worked as a staff supervisor in a home for the developmentally disabled. There was a very sweet man with Down's syndrome there by the name of Ronny. Every night it was Ronny's job to set the table for dinner. He would only set the table at 5:00, not 4:59 and definitely not 5:01. One night when we had an outing planned, the staff and I turned all of the clocks in the house back an hour, so 5:00 would come a little sooner. All was well until we asked Ronny to set the table. He

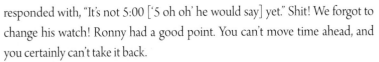

responded with, "It's not 5:00 ['5 oh oh' he would say] yet." Shit! We forgot to change his watch! Ronny had a good point. You can't move time ahead, and you certainly can't take it back.

How different it was to go to bed that night than it was to wake up that very morning. It is so true that you have nothing unless you have your health. How stupid I feel for having complained about the small stuff. Who gives a shit if the kids miss the bus or there are clothes all over my daughter's floor? I have CANCER. Nothing else matters. Now the planner in me needs to come out and I need to make a plan to get through this.

I get a call the next day from Debra, a nurse at the health center. Little did I know during that first conversation, but she would turn out to be one of my Rocks of Gibraltar. She calls me to ask if I have chosen a surgeon and an oncologist yet. WHAT? Jesus, aren't we only 99 percent sure it's cancer? I sat in my basement office holding the phone to my ear in a complete daze. Every ounce of stress permeated my toes all the way through my entire body, leaving me with a pulsing in my head that was hard to ignore. How do you even pick a surgeon? Or better yet, an oncologist? Who the hell would I know? No one. She recommends a surgery group to me and tells me we can talk about it when I go in tomorrow for my biopsy. Thank god I have someone to do the thinking, because it certainly isn't me.

I've never been fascinated by the site of a needle: knitting, hypodermic or otherwise. You'll never catch me in a rocking chair slamming out an itchy wool sweater with a couple of knitting needles, nor will I be first in line for a flu shot. But now the tides are turning, with the surf about to deliver me on a bed of needles.

All I can think about on my way to my biopsy is that I am having a "bibopsy" today. I picture the woman in *My Big Fat Greek Wedding* telling the story of her bibopsy. "They found teeth and a spinal cord. Yes, it twas … my twin." Gotta find some humor here or I'm going to freak. I have an array of amazing friends in my life, many of whom take on the task of being my partner in crime for the many doctor visits I have to endure, the "bibopsy" being the first. My dear friend Jill comes into the office with me as Debra goes over the procedure.

The gist of it is they stick this long-ass needle through your breast and then this vacuum cleaner-type machine sucks the tissue out through the needle. Fun stuff, huh? Of course, I'm asking a million questions, far in advance of what I am having done at that moment. Such as, "What happens next? Will I have to have my breasts removed? If so, do I lose everything?" God bless Debra because she answers every one of my questions. When I ask her about mastectomies, she tells me that sometimes they try to save your nipples and of course, I ask how? Well, how can I put this ... she informs me that sometimes they are removed and attached to your stomach area so they "stay alive," and then they are re-attached to the breast area at a later date.

Again with the "You're shitting me!" That's attractive. With my belly button, it will look like a smiley face! I could pierce my nipples and have a chain going from each nipple to my navel! We laughed so hard—just the thought of it!

The "bibopsy" is like having a needle stuck up your nose and pulled out your ass. It is not pleasant. I count ceiling tiles in order to keep my wits about me. I think if I had the choice, I would give birth again instead of having this needle pressed through my breast. At least I would have something at the end. Another go at a poopy, crying, colicky baby might beat the outcome of this.

Oh, who am I kidding?

I remember leaving the hospital after the birth of my daughter. Derek, my now ex-husband, brought the car seat in, and the nurse made sure my daughter was secure in the seat before we left. I can close my eyes and visualize the little pink outfit, her head to one side looking as if she is being choked by the belt, and the nurse saying, "Looks like you're all set. Let's wheel you out front. Dad, bring the car around." What? No oral or written exam? We can just TAKE her? Well, I'm still figuring this one out, so I'm guessing there's no guide to having cancer either.

While I lay there waiting for the vacuum action to ensue, I chuckle (inside, of course) at an incident from my childhood where my mother tried to invent this very thing. Only, it wasn't cancer cells she was trying to extract, but ear wax. I was about 10 years old and I couldn't hear very well out of my right ear. My mother, being the die-hard nurse that she was, had peered in my ear to discover a blockage of ear wax. I know— gross. But the real comedy of the situation was that my mother had read in one of her "mom magazines," that if you rip up a sheet, wrap a piece around a knitting needle (you can understand my loathing of the needle now), and dip it in wax to harden, you will create an ear wax extracting contraption. Oh, did I mention that the narrow end went into my ear and the other was lit with fire—yes FIRE— to draw out the wax?

To accurately paint the scene, my mother had me lay my head down on the kitchen table, then inserted her contraption, lit the other end and proceeded to leave me there while she went down to the basement to throw in a load of wash. And just as I was thinking, "If anyone could see this—" the flame drew closer and closer to my head and my mom was nowhere to be found. "Oh my god, my hair is going to catch on fire!" I remember thinking. I screamed for my mother and she got there just before the flame hit my hair. Kudos to Mom for thinking outside of the box—but yeah, not the best move.

I'm thinking that my current extraction procedure isn't the best move either, but what choice do I have? I need to know where I stand with this cancer business. I try not to think of where it is or how far along I am in the stages. I will deal with that later. Right now, I need to focus on getting an answer to my question. Do I REALLY have breast cancer? I'm a rational person. I like to see things in black and white. I'm just hoping that this mess isn't going to lead to a pink slip from my life.

Of course, the old adage "two is better than one" applies here, as the doctor found not one, but two suspicious spots to biopsy. The second spot is farther in. JOYOUS! The needle probes yet even further through my breast. Damn, I think I have counted these ceiling tiles twice! Hey, is that a spider in the corner? I focus so hard on that spot that I think there must be a family of spiders up there. Only later do I find out that it was, in fact, just a spot. Well, the spider imagery made the time pass a bit more tolerably. Did I mention that I DON'T live in Crazyville? Yet …

Waiting for test results is always a harrowing experience. Almost like waiting for your SAT scores so you can compare with your friends and see who's got the best chance to make something of themselves. Only to find out twenty five years later than no one gives a rat's ass what you got on your SAT's, just that you did your best and actually became something. Unfortunately, the rating of a cancer test has a purely different outcome. Not "Which college will I attend?", but "Will I have a lumpectomy" or "Will I have my breast removed?" Not "Will I study biology?" but "Will I become the latest cancer biology experiment?"

I endure the longest weekend of my life … waiting. Your mind can become your worst enemy when battling with an unknown. The endless cycle of thoughts becomes even more exhausting than the hamster wheel you may continuously run on. The cage walls, whether plastic or metal grating, come closer and closer to you until, at some point, you realize the only access you have to the outside is your nose and maybe an arm that reaches out, but touches nothing. No answers, only questions.

How do I shut my mind off? I try to imagine a beautiful beach with the surf lapping my feet as I walk. Then an image of my boyfriend lying on the beach "finding himself" pops into my head, and then I just get pissed. Men are the most selfish creatures on the planet. "Me, me, me." I don't mean to speak for all women, but I do believe we have a tendency to think of others more than we think of ourselves. Finding a man who shares this mindset is proving to be quite elusive. My mind goes to Chuck Woolery and the *Love Connection*. God, if only it was that easy. Here are your three choices. One of them is your dream guy. Where is Chuck when I need some guidance?

The fact that he does not fly home immediately to be with me is a huge red flag. Just one that I didn't wanted to deal with at the time. Worse yet, I couldn't face it. We had dated years ago, before I was ever married to Derek. We met up again after all those years, so I have this stupid fairy tale imagery clouding my normally sane thought processes. God, I am such an idiot! Who am I to think that there can be a fairy tale ending in my future?

I remember years earlier walking down the aisle to marry Derek thinking, "What am I doing?" I was 28, almost 29, successful in my career in the family business, always coined the "cute" girl. What was I doing? I wanted a family. I wanted to be somebody's mother. To pass on all of the wonderful things my mother had given me: love, acceptance, belief in myself. It's amazing how the choices we make form us into the individuals we become. Should I have married Dr. Jekyll? In the all-knowing hindsight? Probably not. But I have two incredibly wonderful children that I would not have the privilege to mother had it not been for their father.

An early clue that my marriage was not a match made in heaven came early on with a trip Derek took to the grocery store. It was before we were married on a night I thought I was channeling Betty Crocker and was going to cook up this extraordinary meal that would be showcased on the cover of *Woman's Day* magazine. Needless to say, the meal was terrible but the story would live on as something that should have been a short story in *Reader's Digest.*

He was taking FOREVER, and I remember thinking, where the hell IS he? After what seemed an interminable amount of time waiting, I decided to call. "I'm trying to find a line to check out," he said.

"What do you mean TRYING to find a line?"

To which he responded, "Well, I can't go in the ten items or less line because I have eleven items and I can't go in the 'candy free' aisle."

So, my thinking maybe he had some crazy candy obsession I hadn't yet discovered asked, "Why can't you go in the 'candy free' aisle?"

"Because I have a bag of Starburst." I don't think I stopped laughing for hours. Years later, as my frustration with my marriage mounted, I often reflected on the Starburst incident, knowing that must have been my "sign," but laughed about it anyway.

Only now, I wasn't laughing, and I wasn't crying either. My emotions as flat as my chest is about to become. Thanksgiving quickly approaches, and even though I am paralyzed with fear of my future, I take time to reflect on what I am thankful for. My children, of course. My mother died of breast cancer when I was 26. The pain of that, so raw. I am forever thankful for the time I did have with her. Her life, so impactful on mine and so many others. She had no idea the legacy she would leave. I wonder what legacy will I leave my children. They are seven and eight years old. If I can't beat this, will they even remember me?

Nothing is as scary as looking your own mortality in the face—staring it down and trying to figure out how you can conquer it as quickly as possible. My mother always told me: "You are the master of your own destiny." What now? I'm no longer in control. Something else is. Not someone, but something. It's not as though I can bitch someone out for my failure to live or be well. It's not like I can walk up to Lucy Brown's "The Doctor Is In" and say what the hell is going on here, Lucy? Even Linus and his stupid blanket can't help me out of this mess. I'm feeling more and more like Pigpen—the stinky kid in the sandbox that no one wants to play with—because they don't know what's wrong with me. And so the wait continues through the weekend. Will I play alone in the sandbox?

My father and his wife Gail are on their way up from Florida to experience my wonderful Thanksgiving cooking. I'm not a TERRIBLE cook. Hell, I can READ! If you can read, you can follow a recipe, right? I am so excited for them to come up, for the holiday. Not for my cancer mess.

They arrive at my house, and my father is visibly tormented by what lies ahead for me, for all of us. The years of my mother's struggle to survive is written all over his face. I feel as though he can't even look at me. Like the pain of the past has catapulted to the present and the pain is just too hard to bear. I feel sorry for him. Not in a pitiful way, but so sorry that I am the one to bring this pain back. And then I think wait—I'M THE ONE WITH CANCER! This is MY struggle! Everyone will be watching it from the outside and I will be the one living it. Living the day to day struggle, whatever it will be, will be mine alone.

Monday finally comes after many hours of tormenting mental time. I'm still on a mission to find my own off switch. It would make this whole mess seem more bearable if only to shut it off for a few hours a day. The news comes. Debra calls and tells me that the two spots biopsied are both malignant. One invasive, one non-invasive. I don't even hear the rest. I just hear malignant. And in those poignant moments you only see in made-for-TV movies, I hold the phone away for a moment and take the longest breath of my life. Breathe, Connie. Breathe.

My dad and Gail are downstairs. I have to tell them. I remember the moment my foot hit the top of the stairs. The weight of my legs reminds me of when my kids were little and each held on as I walked. Only no giggles come from down below as I walk. Just a heaviness I have never experienced. Something deadly is running through my body and I want it out. I almost feel dirty. As if a "cleansing" or a colonic will alleviate the weightiness I feel. My foot finally hits the last step and the outcome is written all over my face. But the piss and vinegar side of me that always seems to prevail says, "I cannot fucking believe that this is my life!" Oh my God. Was that my out-loud voice? Did I just say the f-word in front of my father? I look at his face, and yup, it was my out-loud voice. I wait a moment and then realize, I am thirty-nine years old. If I want to say the f-word, I CAN. And really, WHO CARES? I have cancer. CANCER! If ever the f-word is ever warranted, it is now.

My indoor voice chants fuck, FUCK, FUCK as I walk back upstairs to call my boyfriend with the news as he lies on a beach in St. Thomas. I know I sound totally bitter about it, and I don't mean to be. But I do know this. If the person I loved was dealt a terrible blow, I would be on a plane no matter my original plan. I know at that moment and many more to come, where I stand in that love triangle of Mark, me and Mark. Mark and Mark would eventually prevail and I will at some point, months later, come to grips with it.

I call Derek to inform him of my short-term impending doom. I realize (god help me) that I am going to need his help in the coming months with the kids. More importantly, I need to discuss with him how we as parents will break this news to our children. I should know by now, after many years of being married and dealing with flat affect from my ex, that, "Yeah, you'll be OK," in response to my news, is exactly what I should have expected. Nothing more, nothing less. The nothing more grew to include a call back a few minutes later requesting that I "make sure" my life insurance policy names him as the executor to distribute the money to our children. As always, Derek doesn't disappoint. He is probably thinking a payout from my untimely death will be more likely than him ever winning the lottery. I am so far beyond disgusted that there are no words. None. Just a feeling of relief that I don't have to look at his face across the kitchen table day in and day out for the rest of my life. However long or short that life might be. We do, however, decide that I will tell the kids the news when the time is right. I hope that my heart and head come together to form the words for that conversation.

Chapter 2
The Breast Men

*W*hile at my biopsy the week before, Debra had called on my behalf and set up an appointment for me with a general surgeon and a plastic surgeon, my beloved "breast men." She also set up an appointment for me to have an MRI to assess the overall cancer damage. Had it spread to my lymph nodes? The MRI would give my breast surgeon an indication if it had spread.

I have never had an MRI. My son, as an infant, had to have one, and I remember sitting in the room with him while the onslaught of machine gun sounds deafened me. You'd think if a hospital had to spend millions of dollars on a machine such as this, it would find a way to make the damn thing quiet! So here I am, getting my own MRI. I am as close to being claustrophobic as one could be without needing a Xanax to cope. Good thing it is an open-ended MRI or I may have needed multiple doses of anti-anxiety meds.

Again, on with the hospital gown. A male nurse comes over to put my IV in. I HATE needles. As I sit there, I have a defeatist moment when the realization hits me that this is only the beginning of the needle action. There will be so many needles in my future, I will become a human pin cushion sans the felt outer layer. I tell the nurse that I recently had a biopsy and that there are markers in my breast where the tumors are located. I have visions of these little metal things pulled out of me by the magnet from the MRI. A virtual blood bath of breast tissue decorating the noisy machine. At least then, I think, the décor would match the sounds of war emanating from the machine with each picture.

He assures me there will be no problems. He instructs me to lie face down with my breasts each in a hole specifically engineered for optimal breast imagery. You're kidding me, right? It reminds me of those wooden carnival cut-out type things where the face and arms are cut out and you put your own in and wave to the camera. Instead of my face beaming and arms waving at the camera, it's a titty photo op.

The sound of gunfire commences and the imagery is well under way. I lie there in the most awkward of poses, my IV arm over my head, the tubing attached to the IV pole. The nurse clutches the IV post and says, "You're doing great sweetie. Just a few more pictures." Sure, slick. Your tits aren't hanging down in a mold. When is this going to be over?

The MRI finally ends and again, I will have to wait for results. My mother always used to tell me that having cancer is like being in the army. "Hurry up and wait." First of all, what my mother would know about being in the army, I do not know. If she ever had to step foot in an army barracks, she would demand that every man turn over his whites and his handkerchiefs, and then she would make me iron them. Every Saturday morning when I was a kid, I helped my mother iron. Good god! She made me iron my father's handker-chiefs and all I could think about while I ironed was, "My father blows his nose in this thing over and over. Yuck! Doesn't he know someone invented tissues for that very purpose?"

I digress. Yes, my mother had a point. You do hurry up and wait. The reality is that the hurrying takes way more time than the word connotes. The testing seems to take FOREVER, thus far in the process anyway. The waiting, well that's a whole other story. The waiting is cumbersome. Almost like the last few months of pregnancy when you feel like you might explode. With that comes the fear: "Will I be a good mother? Will I know what to do when she cries?" As opposed to this new waiting I am experiencing. "Will I need chemotherapy? Will I be OK?" These latter thoughts drive my mind into a quiet frenzy. There is no outlet. Only more waiting.

My first "breast man" visit is with Dr. B, my breast surgeon. The "removal" guy. I am told by Debra and other nurses at the health center, that not only is he an amazing surgeon, he is great eye candy as well. I figure, hell, if I'm going to have to go through all of this, I might as well have something good to look at.

My father and Gail accompany me to the surgeon's office to find out my fate. I can tell you that before we even get there, whatever options he presents, I am having both of my "girls" removed. Like the burn marks on toast that you scrape off to rid yourself of the taste, I will do the same to my cancer. No bad cancer aftertaste. I will have none of it.

I ask Dad and Gail to wait in the waiting room while I am seen. Dr. B walks in and yes, Debra was right. Eye candy for the masses. Unlike most surgeons and their matter-of-fact mentalities, Dr. B is so caring and kind as he apprises me of my circumstances after my examination. We chat for a bit and he agrees that with my family history, my best option is for a bilateral mastectomy. My MRI showed no lymph node involvement, which is a real positive. He tells me that the mastectomies will be 95 percent of my recovery. Instead of thinking, "Oh great!" my methodical mind is churning over the other 5 percent. What is that going to be? Well, I will find out soon enough.

I ask my father and Gail to come into the room to speak with the surgeon. My father breaks down and sobs in front of the surgeon. I have yet to shed a tear since my diagnosis with Chatty Cathy and the radiologist. I have no tears, just disbelief and agony over what is yet to come. All I keep thinking is "God, he has to pull himself together or I'm going to have to bitch-slap him." I understand his fear, concern and ever-apparent pain over this, but I make a mental note to speak with my stepmother about this. It can't go on. I am having a hard enough time keeping myself together for me, let alone my kids. I can't keep myself together for anyone else.

My next meeting is with my plastic surgeon. Because of the nature of this visit, and that of my mind, I ask my friend Amy to accompany me on this adventure because she is one of my funny friends. A friend I can look at with a raised eyebrow and laughter will undoubtedly ensue. As we walk into the doctor's waiting room, this man with a white coat and Kramer-type wild hair walks past us into the office. Is that the doctor? OK, if Alan Funt is dead, he must have a son carrying on the family business, no?

15

We waltz into the examining room. Me, ready for the next onslaught of news to come. The nurse, Kari, who I will later love for her sense of humor and knack of keeping my doctor in check, comes in to get a history. She asks me how many children I have and how old they are. I tell her they are seven and eight. Her response, as is that of so many others: "Wow, that's close." When I am nervous or stressed, my humor comes to the forefront as sketchy sarcasm. To her comment, I reply, "Yeah, I couldn't keep my knees together." She laughs and I immediately feel at ease.

She leaves me and Amy alone to meander through a photo album of before and after shots. A far cry from the before and after beauty shots I used to take as a Mary Kay Beauty Consultant and Sales Director. No, these were not glamour shots at all. Quite the contrary. No head shots, just-below-the-neck shots of women's breasts. The before and after fakeness that I have yet to personally experience. Nipples; no nipples. Scars and more scars. We see a woman in a photo with a pearl necklace. Amy and I decide to call her the pearl necklace chick. Her before and after looks appear satisfactory to me. The other photos are all of older women. You can tell by the slump of the shoulders and the sag of the before breasts that they are older. The slump of the shoulders looks like an admittance of defeat. Pearl necklace chick has her shoulders squared, like an "I take no shit from cancer" stance not to be messed with. I will remember this stance for my before and after shots.

Kari comes back to describe the reconstruction process. She tells me over and over that I don't have to do it now (at the time of my mastectomies). I can opt to do it later on. I will tell you that after experiencing it, I now see why they give you the option. We talk about nipple reconstruction. Because of the invasiveness of my cancer, I'm not one of the "lucky" ones who gets to have my nipples transplanted to my abdomen for future reattachment. I will not only become a tit-less wonder, but a nipple-less tit-less wonder!

I have been so upset about this, the thought of losing my nipples. Before I was diagnosed, I would think, "What's the big deal about breasts anyway?" Well, for one, they make us look like women. However, they do not MAKE us women. I always struggled with THO's (titty hard ons) as coined by my college girlfriends, when it was cold out and we had the involuntary reaction to the cold weather. Or, as my friend Angela calls it, "Nippleopolis." Since finding out I would lose my nipples, I had recurring dreams of myself getting out of the shower and passing by my bathroom mirror. No signs of redness on my chest, just a flesh-colored front that caused me to wake up in a sweat, pinching myself to confirm that this was now my reality.

I think back to a nipple incident a few years back when I had to go to a work function in Maine at my then-company's headquarters. I was never into padded bras. Plain and simple, it was the itch factor. I wore a white dress shirt, with an obvious non-padded bra. It was November I think. It was cold, but not the cold where you wanted to wear a bulky winter coat. I traveled to the function with two of my coworkers, Julie and Claire. We walked into this boardroom for a meeting. Of course, we were the only women. I remember thinking, "Why is everyone staring at me? Do I look THAT fabulous?" During a break in the meeting, the three of us traipsed over to the ladies' room, me the last one to enter. "HOLY MOTHER OF GOD!" I yelled.

Julie and Claire said, "What's the matter?"

I pointed at the mirror and said, "Look!" And there, in my reflection, were my nipples, showing through my white blouse as big as saucers! No wonder I was so popular that afternoon! I gather up a scarf from someone and wear it over each breast for the remainder of the meeting.

One of my male co-workers later said, "Hey Con, let me see your blouse."

"Bite me," I said as everyone laughed uproariously.

Well, there would be no more nipple incidents. No more THO worries. On the bright side, I might be able to kick some twenty-year-old's ass in a wet t-shirt contest! OK, maybe I shouldn't go that far…

Not only are nipples part of the appearance factor for a woman, but they are also part of our sexual being. If things don't work out with my boyfriend Mark, who will want me with no nipples? Better yet, who will want me after having had breast cancer? If I was still married to Dr. Jekyll, he'd have to deal with my nipple-less self because he would be stuck with me. Who would want to be stuck with me now? For the most part, I have always thought of myself as a secure person. Mark has always commented on how I am comfortable in my own skin. Well, who else's skin could I have? At this point, I am almost willing to switch.

I have three options for nipples after my reconstruction.

One: I could just go without. No more wet t-shirt contest see-through worries. No more THO worries.

Two: I could have them tattooed on. What the hell would that look like? I picture myself being tattooed by the typical tattoo artist. Face piercings and tattoos like "your mama was my bitch" on an arm, all the while leering at my bare chest with his pierced tongue hanging out. "I got myself a plain canvas now!" No thanks. Kari assures me that they have a medical tattoo artist whose tattoo specialty is nipples. I imagine this man showing up at his twenty-year high school reunion. Memories of my own reunion last summer, still visible in my mind. "Bob, so wonderful to see you! What do you do for a living?"

"Well, I did some soul searching trying to figure out where I could really leave my mark in the world. And then, I had a revelation. I decided to become a medical tattoo artist."

"And what is your specialty Bob?"

"Well, I've always considered myself a titman so I am a nipple tattoo artist."

Good grief! My imagination is taking me to some scary places.

Option three: nipple reconstruction. And what might that entail? Inquiring minds want to know. How can I put this delicately? They take skin from your labia—yeah that's right, down there—and make it into a nipple. As Forrest Gump would say, "Life is like a box of chocolates. You never know what you're gonna get!" The same would apply to the outcome of the nipple reconstruction, or dare I say, the labia-octomy. You have to be kidding me. The next man who decides to nibble on me will be nibbling not a nipple, but a point down yonder masquerading as a nipple. Good news for all those boys who want a home run sooner rather than later.

Oh my god, what is happening to me? How can this possibly be? My next life-changing decision is what cup size I want to be. Well, if you're going to have "store-boughts" they might as well be spectacular, right? I opt for a size up, of course. A C cup it will be! Kari shows me what the expander is and how it works. The expander is placed between your rib cage and your chest muscle. Oh yes, people. Now that I am through all of this, I can confidently flex my chest muscles like Sean Astin in 50 First Dates.

The expander looks like a flattened implant. Thicker plastic that puckers around the edges, which subsequently end up feeling sharp in your chest. I know nothing at this point about the sharpness factor, so I just listen to Kari as she tells the story of how I will come in weekly, and Dr. R (yes, Kramer) will insert a needle and add saline volume to my chest until I get to a point where I am comfortable. Once that is accomplished, I will have a surgery to remove the expanders and implant my new tatas and that will be the end of the breast story. Well, almost.

Chapter 3
Lobbing Off

*M*y surgery is scheduled in two weeks' time because both surgeons have to coordinate their schedules so I can have everything done at one time. Two weeks to think about everything. Two weeks of a mental death sentence. To sit and ponder my fate, not knowing the outcome. Yes, I will get new breasts, but will I need chemotherapy? My best hope is that I will have everything removed, get new boobs, do the dreaded tattooed nipple bit and be done with this mess.

My friends encourage me to start a *Caring Bridge* website so that I will not receive a million phone calls about my cancer. The barrage of "How are you feeling?" questions can be assuaged with a blog-type venue where people can read about my progress. Done. I'm cool with that, and it was a great release for me to write down my story, as I am now.

I choose a password for others to access my site and think "fortitude" to be most fitting under the circumstances. I start the site and see that I must write my "story." I've always been a firm believer in the "keep it short and sweet," so here it is:

Background Story

> I am so grateful for the love and support of my family and
> friends. Without all of you, this journey would be much
> more difficult. As most of you know, my mother lost her

battle with breast cancer twelve years ago at the age of fifty-three. And even though I have been prepared for this diagnosis on some level, it has certainly taken the wind from my sails. Alyssa and Alex, at eight and seven, need their mom to be her crazy spastic self. This is a small bump in the road. My prognosis is good. We caught it early. I will survive this for my children and for my mother, who never got the opportunity to beat it. Thank you all again for your thoughts and prayers.

What else do I say? I have nothing else. I have wasted hours of brain time on my future, whatever it was to be.

My gynecologist calls me and says, "Connie, I am so sorry. This is going to be a very tough year for you." And here I was thinking, just a few months. Little did I know at that point that the journey is ongoing. That you can relieve yourself of the physical cancer, but the rest of it remains.

My friends write messages on my *Caring Bridge* site. How amazing it is for me to read these and be inspired to keep going, even though this is just the beginning.

Monday, December 8, 2008 2:55 PM, CST

Connie my sweet friend, know that I am with you in spirit when you go in for surgery along with all who love and adore you. You are loved more than you know! I will be in contact and please know that I am here for you in any way that you need. You are an inspiration to all. Your strength and spirit are incredible. I love you with all my heart and soul!

Deana

Monday, December 8, 2008 3:00 PM, CST

Connie, I can't tell you how humbled I have been with your incredibly positive attitude and outlook over the past several weeks. All of your friends here in the Wild West may be miles away but we are with you in heart. I won't say be strong because we already know that you are!

Doug

Monday, December 8, 2008 3:20 PM, CST

Dear Connie - I am sorry to hear what you are going through. I can hear in your words how positive and strong you sound! Best of luck on Wednesday and hope you are feeling better really soon!

Lisa G.

Monday, December 8, 2008 3:41 PM, CST

Connie,

I was shocked to learn (about 5 minutes ago) that you have breast cancer and are about to go in for surgery. I wish I could do something to help. You are so brave and have such positive energy…I know you'll come through it just fine. Still wish I could make the path a bit easier. Good luck on Wednesday and know that you are loved and my thoughts (and many others) are with you.

Love,

Linda Z.

Monday, December 8, 2008 4:26 PM, CST

Connie, you are in my thoughts and prayers. I will be especially thinking of you on Wed. and sending lots of positive energy your way. You are so strong and resilient. I am sorry you have to go through this but I know you will come through it stronger than ever. I am here to help in any way—please let me know if you need anything in the upcoming weeks.

Love,

Mary Beth F.

Monday, December 8, 2008 4:57 PM, CST

Connie, you have been in my thoughts since we spoke last week. I am sorry that you need to go through this and I wish with all my heart it wasn't true. Looking forward to knowing that in just a few days you'll be on the road to recovery. Sending love your way and I promise I'll make you laugh when you need to!

Joan F.

Monday, December 8, 2008 5:27 PM, CST

COONNNNSTANCE!!!!!

You know I love you babe you rock chick you're incredible :) Call me if you need help with anything!!!! I love you to death and can't wait for the end of this chapter for you!!!

Andrea G.

Monday, December 8, 2008 6:20 PM, CST

Connie,

Wow...I had no idea! Be strong, which we both know you can do, be brave, you can do it girl and beat this thing... your mom is watching over you and will help you thru it.

Have faith, between your faith, your love, and your friends and family...you will do fine. I will pray for you, and will anxiously await news after the surgery...God Bless you. Hugs and Love Nancy D.

Monday, December 8, 2008 8:55 PM, CST

Connie

I will be thinking and praying for you on Wednesday and wish you a quick recovery. You're a very strong person and will get through this. I am here for you and available to help in anyway I can. You are in my thoughts and prayers.

With love,

Chris P.

Tuesday, December 9, 2008 8:30 AM, CST

Connie,

I am so sorry to hear this. My mom and grandmother had breast cancer and my grandma passed away from it as she let it go too long before getting diagnosed, but my mom is a survivor. I will keep you and your family in my thoughts and prayers for all to go well! Keep up your positive energy!!!

Wendy C.

Tuesday, December 9, 2008 2:14 PM, CST

Cone,

As I sit here thinking about what you are about to endure, the right words are hard to find.

We have been friends for a LONG TIME (before kindergarten, right?), and you have NEVER backed down from a challenge. I know you will be able to close this chapter in your life shortly and get on with things.

I am always just a phone call away, so don't hesitate to call for anything. Even if you just want to laugh; I've got a few things you may have forgotten but I remember! :)

Love always,

Juan (John P)

Tuesday, December 9, 2008 2:52 PM, CST

Connie,

You are one of the strongest women that I know. I feel with all my heart you will beat this thing and come out even better, if that is possible. Keep your positive outlook, it is contagious. We are all pulling for you.

Love ya

Kellie H.

Tuesday, December 9, 2008 7:20 PM, CST

Hey Sweetie!!!

Always thinking of you!! You really are an inspiration to us all with your positive attitude and incredible strength. Whatever I can do, I will be right there. Love you lots xoxoxox Jill

Over the next two weeks, my head is in all sorts of places. I imagine my mother after her own mastectomy. The whiteness of her skin, the defeat in her expression. Remembering the feeling I had seeing her like that.

Will my children look at me and see the same thing in me? What if the cancer has spread into my lymph nodes? After all, my last mammogram, not a year before, showed nothing. How invasive is this cancer? Invasive enough to dictate my future physicality, but surely not my future mentality. Or is it?

I sit my kids down to tell them about my surgery. I may not be able to control all of what is yet to come, but I can control how I react to it and how I portray it to my kids. My children, the loves of my life. I will not tell them that I have cancer, not yet. They know what it is. We've talked about it. They know that people die from it. I know that if I say the C-word, it will open up a proverbial can of worms that right now I can't deal with. Those worms would inevitably divide until there were too many to catch, the can overflowing, and too many questions left unanswered.

I tell them that I am OK, but I need to have an operation.

"What for?" Alex, my seven year old asks.

"Well, my doctor found something on my chest that he doesn't like, so he is going to remove it and I will be all better." I tell them about the tubes that will come out of my chest and how for a few weeks they won't be able to squeeze me tight when they hug me.

My daughter takes on a thoughtful expression and says, "OK." Is it that easy? Do they buy everything I tell them? Of course they do! I'm their mother! I've never ever given them a reason not to believe what I have to say. I will be better, I think. At least I hope so. If not, I will cross that bridge when I come to it and not a day sooner.

I go back and forth over these next two weeks between thoughts of my own mortality and feelings of failure over my fairy tale ending with the prince. He went off to St. Thomas for a month to "find himself," well, because he could. He worked his tail off with his company, realized there was more to life at the age of forty-three, and went about seeking those answers. I don't blame him for his choices. He is who he is and no matter where we are at in our lives I will always love him. But he wasn't there for me when I needed him to be and therein lies the realization of my future with the would-be prince. I knew then my fate in the fairy tale. The fairy tale would end with me walking away from the prince and his castle, a future unknown in love and in life. For the meantime though, I will meander through and take from it what I can because, well, I loved him. Love makes you do stupid things and allows your heart to put up with things that in a love sobered mind you would not be so tolerant.

Mark came back from St. Thomas the night before my surgery. He came to my house the next morning, almost a month having passed since we had last seen each other, to take me to my dreaded day of surgery. My hair was shorter—I had a bob and upon word of my surgeries and possibly not being able to shower for two weeks (good god!), I decided to cut my hair short. No more flat-ironing and primping for me.

I have visions of myself after my surgeries, wiping myself down with baby wipes and have, in fact, sufficiently supplied myself with some for this adventure. I know I look worn. God knows I feel it. As he opens my car door, I feel a strain in my heart for the last month, in tandem with a relief that my boyfriend/lover/friend will be here for me during this journey.

My brother Kurt comes up from North Carolina to be with me for my surgery and then fly back the following day. My mother would be so proud and pleased about our relationship in adulthood. The days of beating the shit out of each other are over. We are both parents to her never-seen grandchildren and good friends to one another. Ever the comedian, Kurt accompanies us on my sobering ride to the hospital, providing much needed laughter along the way.

I change into the hospital gown, something that will inevitably become a staple to my wardrobe over the next few months. I crack jokes with my doctors, I think trying to put them more at ease with me than me with them. I feel so very small lying there in that bed. Not small and insignificant, but small and almost frail. I am an active woman. I play soccer, I work out, I am strong in business and yet I remember the sense of feeling so small in that moment. Like there was nothing more I could do. My fate was in the hands of other people. A difficult venture for me, the control freak. Little did I know, this day was the beginning of my learning how to live life one day at a time. My thoughts are no longer of who is on my day planner for lunch next Tuesday, but how I will finish out the day.

The anesthesiologist would later become a revered friend during my many surgeries. My provider of "happy juice," making the journey to unconsciousness seem kinder, more peaceful, and at times, even a little giddy. I remember thinking as the "happy juice" was coursing through my IV, that this was my last moment to be whole. That from this moment forward, I would not be my whole self, just a version of myself, missing pieces. Pieces that would later be there, but fraudulent in their being.

I wake up with a heaviness in my chest that I cannot fully describe. In many ways it feels like the proverbial "elephant on the chest," but with a heaviness of a missing link. It's over. At least this part is over, but the journey ahead looks long. And I can deal with long, just as long as I know that a positive outcome will prevail.

Another staple to my wardrobe arrives: the zip-up surgical bra. White, huge and cumbersome, holding what little chest I have tight to my body. It is itchy and annoying and I don't know it then, but I will have to wear this god awful thing for months.

I have three tubes coming out of my chest with grenade-type bulbs on the other end, collecting fluid from my chest. I know, really attractive. I would later make peace with these drains, as I would have more to come. The weight of the fluid in the drains pulls on me and I remember thinking, this shit is not going to fly for long. Mark has the brilliant idea of putting them in a fanny pack. It is pretty brilliant, although the zipper on the damn pack moves every time I walk and after a couple of weeks, I can't stand the sound of my own coming and going.

During my three-night stay in the hospital, the Northeast experiences an incredible ice storm, with power outages everywhere, including my own house. My friends and family call, so I decide it is a great time to start writing in my online journal.

Thursday, December 11, 2008 3:41 PM, CST

Hey Everyone! I am doing great! I will be coming home from the hospital tomorrow. I had an allergic reaction to the pain medicine and have been itchy. Fun stuff! Nothing a bit of Demerol and Darvocet can't fix! Thanks for all of your good thoughts, prayers and messages. If any of you call and I say something stupid, remember I am ON DRUGS! Love to all, Con:)

Thursday, December 11, 2008 8:11 AM, CST

Morning Sunshine,

Hope you had sweet dreams and stopped scratching! SOOOOOOO good to hear your voice. Just thinking of you and sending XXXXXXXXXXOOOOOOOO. Peaceful, Healing thoughts

Laurie K.

Thursday, December 11, 2008 8:46 AM, CST

Con, it's great to hear the surgery went well and you are doing OK. Please let me know if I can do anything at all for you from Texas.

Haley

Thursday, December 11, 2008 10:30 AM, CST

Cone,

Michelle called me yesterday after surgery to give me the news...HUGE RELIEF! Please post on the site when you are ready for visitors...

Juan (John P)

Thursday, December 11, 2008 10:53 AM, CST

WOOOHOOO GIRL—Yet ANOTHER challenge you have successfully conquered. I am soooo proud of you; you have been an inspiration of strength and unbelievable character—my prayers continue as always and I am here for any assistance you may need. Please call if there is anything I can do to help. Connie—please let us know when you feel up for company. Luv ya – Kathy S.

Thursday, December 11, 2008 11:02 AM, CST

Constance,

Your strength and determination is absolutely wonderful and you are an inspiration to those around you. It was great to talk to you and you sound wonderful...of course I would expect no less from you!!!! I love you and know that my prayers for you will continue through all of this.

Love and God Bless you always,

Lisa H. XOXO

Thursday, December 11, 2008 11:48 AM, CST

Dear Connie,

Thank goodness for text messaging though I now have access to my computer again. So glad to hear that the surgery went well and better yet to see that your sense of humor continues to thrive. I am sure you know it will be your humor that gets you through this. I can only imagine the number of friends you have who are anxious to come and visit and the number of phone calls that are just waiting to be made to you. You are loved by every one of us in our own special way.

Just reading some of the notes it's a given you touch us all in a unique way. I've made arrangements for a friend to drop off a few meals starting next week.

Anyway, I will call you when it quiets down and I will drop in from time to time. This is a GREAT website! I love you more than you will ever know.

Love,

Your sister and friend and most of all YOUR OLD BABYSITTER from 36 years ago.

Ellen

Thursday, December 11, 2008 12:35 PM, CST

Connie,

I am so incredibly happy to hear that your surgery was so successful. I cannot wait to talk to you and see you. You are such a wonderful friend to all of us and we are so grateful that the surgery is behind you!!

Much love,

Chris H.

Thursday, December 11, 2008 3:09 PM, CS

Hey there girl, Jim and I are sending our thoughts and prayers, glad to hear you are liking the drugs, I am sure you would just love to share...Lets us know if we can do any-thing...yeah I know we aren't right down the road, but we love road trips...Godspeed...Laura and Jim...

Chapter 4
The Itchy Heal

I t is SO great to read these messages. My friends and family are throwing me life preservers so I don't drown. All of my "lifelines" on *Who Wants To Be A Millionaire* have probably been used up by now, so I am eternally grateful for all of the extras.

While I was in the hospital, I had an allergic reaction to one of the pain medications. I had a rash from ass to elbow. OK, not really, but it was pretty bad. My abdomen, arms, legs and back were completely raw. In hindsight, maybe it was a blessing: to occupy my mind with the itch and not the loss of my breasts.

I feel hideous. My breasts are gone. I am still my happy self, laughing and joking with my family and friends, but at the same time I feel robbed. Much like the bank teller who receives the "put all the money in the bag or else" note. Fork over your tits lady, or you're going to die.

I stay at Mark's house for the weekend following my surgery. He takes amazing care of me, so attentive to my needs. Maybe my fairy tale ending will come to pass. I remember asking him while he was in St. Thomas, if he would be able (and willing) to spend the first week after my surgery sleeping at my house in case I needed something in the night. He assured me he would be there and my brother's wife Melissa (who came up from NC to help) would be here with me during the day.

Thank god I am able to shower (with Melissa on the other side of the curtain to ensure I don't fall and break my ass) and don't have to wash myself down with the copious supply of baby wipes I purchased. I laugh thinking back on all of the wipes I used on my kids. I'm relieved those days are over. I was very protective over the wipe usage when my kids were babies. One Fourth of July weekend, Derek and I took the kids to my hometown to see the parade and stopped for a bite to eat at a restaurant with some friends. Derek went to town wiping his hands with the wipe supply, and I, unbeknownst to me, used my OUTDOOR voice to say, "HEY, take it easy on the wipes! We won't have any to wipe their asses with!"

It is extremely tiring to shower, but hey, it beats the wipe scenario!

Having your breasts removed results in limited arm mobility and a lot of pain. The simplest movements knock the wind out of me. I'm not allowed to lift anything heavier than ten pounds. I'm always on the go doing things, so having limitations is not something I can easily tolerate. I remember when I was pregnant with my daughter, I had pregnancy-induced hypertension and was put on bedrest for the last two weeks before I was finally induced. I was supposed to lie on my left side, only getting up to go to the bathroom. On one occasion, I got up to go to the bathroom and two hours later had cleaned out the bathroom cabinets. Not to mention the fact that I found a stain on the carpet and decided that instead of using spot removal, I would steam vacuum the entire rug. So no, I don't take well to limitations.

My ex-husband took my children during my surgery and for much of that first week. I want to see them so they know that I am OK. I am so afraid of them seeing me in a bad state. In their eyes, I am their strong, crazy, fun mother. What will their reaction be to how I look? Tubes come out of my chest, grenade-like, fluid-holding thingies hang there, held in a fanny pack to my waist. I put a little makeup on, hide the "grenades" in the fanny pack, and think I will put on my happy Mom face even though I am in pain.

I finally come home to my own house. Mark drops me off for a few hours and Derek brings the kids by to see me for awhile. The electricity is back on but it is extremely cold in the house. The kids open the front door and my aching anticipation of their arrival immediately recedes. I am their mother! They will love me no matter how bad I look! We are so happy to see each other. My son, my little love bug, grabs hold of me and I have to tell him to be careful because my chest hurts. My daughter reluctantly gives me a loose hug, tears in her eyes as she says she is afraid she will hurt me. I am tired. I think I am invincible, but even two hours of talking and playing games with my kids tires me beyond anything I had imagined. After many careful hugs and many kisses, they go back with their Dad for the rest of the week. After a few days, I know I will be much stronger. Their old Mom will be back. The crazy lunatic one, who sings songs with them into play microphones. Yeah, her. She'll be back.

Monday, December 15, 2008 10:20 AM, CST

Hi everyone! I finally got home this morning. Because of the power outages, I have been at my boyfriend Mark's house. Thank goodness for fireplaces! It looks like a war zone in my neighborhood. It's pretty shocking to see all of the tree damage.

I feel pretty good, although I feel like I have had a run-in with a Mack truck. I am doing well with the drains in my chest (what chest??) and I have a follow-up with the plastic surgeon tomorrow. On Thursday, I meet with my general surgeon and find out the results of the tissue pathology to see where I go from here. Hopefully, no treatment.

I'm going to take another Darvocet and try to sleep. Thanks for all of your thoughts and prayers. It should be all "uphill" from here. No pun intended:)

Wednesday, December 17, 2008 10:33 AM, CST

Hey chickie…glad you are recuperating fairly well. I hope to get to see you this weekend. I will call to see if you are up to a Saturday visit on Thursday. I know you are strong and will get thru this with flying colors!!! Let me know how and when I can help!!! Love you!!

Jen K.

Wednesday, December 17, 2008 11:36 AM, CST

Hi Connie,

So glad to read your update. Donna called me the day of your surgery to let me know Lisa said you made out OK. By the grace of God, you are getting better and better every day. I pray for your complete and fast recovery. With your attitude and fun spirit, you'll enjoy the holidays with Alex and Alyssa. I know you know that you have LOTS of people who LOVE YOU and are praying for you!

Maureen L.

That first week was grueling. Melissa helped me with laundry, food shopping and just plain getting around. I didn't eat much. Nothing tasted good. I toiled with the thought of investing in Stouffers as the only food I would eat was Stouffers macaroni and cheese. I took about twenty pills per day. Antibiotics, iron, pain, asthma medications— I had to write down a schedule of medications. I almost felt like an elderly person in a home. I think, wow, if I have a hard time keeping all of this shit straight, how do they do it?

And let me tell you about the drains. What a freaking pain in the ass! Three plastic grenade- type appendages that not only hung from my body, but filled with fluid that had to be measured and drained every few hours. Sleeping without leaking all over my clothes and bed became a chore of infinite proportions, much like maneuvering through a mine field. In the dark. With sunglasses on.

Mark never stays with me at night. Any of these nights. Another red flag to add to my flag collection. I know he fights with some issues. I try to be sympathetic, but I have never been in his position, so how do I know? He was having one of his "weeks." Well I was having one of MINE and there is nothing more isolating than actually being alone going through all of this. No pity party needed. It is what it is and I deal with it. Even when I was married, I wouldn't have woken Derek up in the night to tell him what I was thinking and feeling because he would inevitably say some stupid-ass thing that would send me into a tizzy. But it would be nice to know someone was there. Someone I could turn to with all my fear and have him say, "You're going to be OK, baby."

I give Mark carte blanche to walk away. "I will be fine, I have tons of friends," I say. He says he will be there for me because he loves me. I take what I can get and run with it. What else can I do? One part of me thinks I should just end it and deal with the ramifications. I will be heart broken, but I will go on. I will live. No relationship is worth losing yourself over. And yet, I hang in there, ever the lonely one, thinking it will all turn around at some point.

My sister-in-law Melissa takes me to my surgeon for my follow up visit. The thought of having chemotherapy never really enters my mind. I think they've gotten it all and I will get a new rack and all will be well with the world. Nothing prepares me for what I am about to learn.

Chapter 5
Poisons and Other Potions

Thursday, December 18, 2008 7:31 PM, CST

I saw my surgeon today and got my pathology results. I was hoping for better news. I have a micro-metastasis (spelling?) in my lymph nodes. It is about 1mm in size. I am having another surgery on January 9th to remove some (hopefully not all) of my lymph nodes on my left side and having a mediport put in my chest for chemotherapy. My surgeon said I am looking at 6 to 12 months of chemotherapy, but I won't know the total scoop until I meet with my oncologist on the 30th. I am really stunned with this news. I had figured that I would go to his office today, he would say "everything looks good," I would get new boobs and call it a day. Not the case.

I am incredibly thankful for all of my friends and family for their support. My Dad and Gail spent a month up here helping me and taking care of me for which I am completely grateful. They came up for Thanksgiving dinner and my food didn't kill them, so they decided to stay :) My brother's wife Melissa (who is WONDERFUL) flew up from NC on Sunday and has been here with me every day this week taking care of me and yelling at me if I move (kidding). Everyone knows I can't sit down. I'm having a hard time with this, especially the part about resting.

My brother Kurt flew up from NC for my surgery and then went back the day after, which I SO APPRECIATED. He is coming back up tomorrow, so it will be wonderful to spend time him, Melissa and their kids. Kurt has been so good to me. (As he should be because I ROCK as a sister!)

I am going to be OK, but this is going to be a really long haul. I am worried about the kids and upsetting them. They don't know I have cancer at this point. I will somehow have to cross this bridge soon. I know how it felt at 19 to know what my mother was going through. I don't know if it will be harder or easier for them because they are so little. I hope the latter. This is what I am most worried about.

I have already decided that if I lose my hair, I am going to get some kind of a "lunatickish" wild wig. Why not?

Thank you all so much for caring for me and writing all of these amazing messages. To all my friends close by, stop over. I need some laughs! Love to you all, Connie :)

I am so blessed. I have so many friends and a wonderful family. The messages written to me on my *Caring Bridge* site give me the courage and strength to keep my spirits in check.

Thursday, December 18, 2008 4:05 PM, CST

Connie,

I just got off the phone with Jill...please know I am praying and that I will be here for you for your entire journey through this ordeal and beyond.

xo Missy T.

Thursday, December 18, 2008 7:47 PM, CST

Connie,

I think about you every day. Please let me know if you need anything. You have two wonderful kids who have shown their adaptability and perseverance. I know they, and you, are going to come out of this better than fine. My thoughts and prayers are with you and your family.

PS—You would look SO good in some kind of bright pink wig with really long hair. Totally you.

Elena T.

Thursday, December 18, 2008 9:01 PM, CST

Hi Connie,

Talked with Joan today, and we can't wait to come up there and hear some funny stories that only you can tell! I am going to call you to see what might work for you. Thinking about you everyday and lots of prayers too.

xoxo, Britt T.

Thursday, December 18, 2008 10:48 PM, CST

Hi Connie, I was so happy to hear your voice today. I'm so sorry that you didn't hear the words you wanted from your doctor. Remember you have to take one day at a time!!! Let me know when you're up for a visit and if I can help with the kids? You can call me anytime day or night. Many prayers are being said for you to help you on this journey.

Love you lots, Chris F.

Friday, December 19, 2008 8:18 AM, CST

Connie...if you end up needing a wig, you should definitely get a purple one!! LOL

Love ya—Kate D.

Kate D.

Friday, December 19, 2008 8:25 AM, CST

Hey You,

No soft and mushy sentiments from me other than THIS REALLY FRIGGIN BLOWS!!!!!!! Anyway, uphill we go again; no problem as we are a couple of tough broads!! Although I am down here in Brewster I can be there in 2 hours, just call and I mean ANYTIME!!! As my sister from another mother I will give you nothing less then 100%. From my own experiences, the children are resilient and will process what they can. Remember our talk yesterday morning, they love you for you and nothing will touch that perfect bond. I was thinking a mohawk of various shades and some tattoos on either side of it would be outstanding for the new year. I love you to the moon and stars and back!!!!! xoxoxox Laurie K.

Friday, December 19, 2008 1:48 PM, CST

Hi Connie,

I didn't expect to hear your news either...thought it would be clear sailing from here, but this too, shall pass. It is but another bump that will show you more blessings especially when it looks like the opposite. It is so nice to hear about your family being all around you. How great is that? OK, so now on to the next hurdle and with your kids…they don't need to know more than they can handle…which is only simple, brief words with encouragement that you will still be here for them…and you will.

I will continue to pray and wait to hear from you…Love, Anna B.

Words cannot express the defeat I feel leaving that doctor's office. What a devastating blow! Six to twelve months of chemo. OMG! How am I going to survive that? How am I going to work and support my kids as a single mother? Better yet, how am I going to physically survive all of it while pasting on a happy mother face day after day for my kids?

Melissa and I get in the car and I am speechless. That, and I was just plain pissed off. How could it have gotten this far? I was on top of my health. I had mammograms every year! I am only thirty-nine years old! WTF! I have Melissa call my dad and Gail. I just can't talk to anyone. I don't want to face all of the questions. I don't have any answers, so what is the point? How do I tell my kids that they are going to have a bald mother? A very sick bald mother?

As we drive home, I stare out the window at all of the white and deadness that is winter. I feel the same as the nothingness I am looking at. I close my eyes and will myself to another place. Lost in my thoughts, I find myself on a plane going somewhere. Any place but here. The g-force of takeoff throws me back in my seat and I stare out the window at blackness. There is no light, only flickers of yellow and red beneath me. I look for the horizon, but don't see it. It is too dark. What am I looking for? I realize at that moment, that what I am searching for is within ME, nothing I can find outside of myself. I snap open my eyes and look out at the sparse trees of the season. We share the same anatomy. The easy spirit of green has faded, and so have I.

I arrive home and go down to the basement. My company has been so good to me. I work from home, which is a complete godsend, especially with the battle that is before me. Down in the basement are the flowers they sent after my surgery. A dozen stargazer lilies. The very flower I abhor for its smell and the reminder of my mother's mortality. I remember the funeral home smell hitting my nose as I descended the stairs to meet the flowers face-to-face. Ever since the day of my mother's funeral, that smell has a way of evoking tears even under the happiest of circumstances. That flower, so pretty and light, signifies a heaviness that I can't escape. I remember sitting on the couch in my basement looking at the flowers as they stared back at me from the coffee table. I will make peace with these flowers. It is time. It is my time to make a choice.

My mother always told me that life was for the living. And live I will. I will embrace this flower not for the loss its smell reminds me of, but for the life I will live in spite of all of life's obstacles. This cancer will not get the best of me. I pick up the vase, bring it upstairs and put it on my dining room table. Melissa says, "I thought you hated those flowers. Why did you bring them upstairs?" I tell her I made peace with them. She meets my gaze with a raised eyebrow.

It's her own fault for marrying into this family, right?

I am off of work for a week and a half. Now it is time to go back to the daily grind. Like I said, I work from home, which proves to be invaluable at this time. I prop pillows up in my bed, laptop on my lap, pain pills on my nightstand and I get back to work. I fall easily back into work. I am a product trainer for a company in the automotive industry. I spend a lot of time on the phone, much of the time spent conducting webinar training sessions. Simply put, I need to be on top of my game, so I opt to hold off on the narcotic pain pills while I'm working. This proves to be a challenge as I grit my teeth a bit while I work that first week.

Chapter 6
Hope and Holly

*T*he Christmas holiday is approaching. It is Derek's turn to have Christmas with the kids. I ask to have them for a couple of hours on Christmas Day, because my brother is here for the holidays, but he refuses. Another ongoing battle that I just don't have the energy to fight. I spent the two weeks prior to my surgery Christmas shopping for both of the kids, wrapping the presents and putting them in a box for Derek to take to his apartment, so he would have no worries for the kids at Christmas. And I can't have two hours with my children on Christmas Day? When my brother and his family are here? When I have breast cancer? I have no words other than to say that this is a recurring theme in my relationship with my ex-husband. A theme that, after this life-changing event, I have little to no tolerance for.

Tuesday, December 23, 2008 3:00 PM, CST

> Hey Everyone! I am doing really well. My drains were taken out this morning, so I am feeling human again (well, almost)! I am on my way with Mark to Connecticut to spend Christmas with his family. He has been so wonderful to me and his family is great so I am really looking forward to spending the holidays with them. The kids are with their

Dad for Christmas, so we will be celebrating Christmas this weekend when I get them back. Alex thinks it's the coolest thing that Santa comes to two places for him. I meet with my oncologist next Tuesday to really find out the scoop about the chemo situation. I am doing really well. All of you, my friends and family, have been amazing to me. I'm still my spastic self. Probably more so than usual. I am on so many medications, I almost ACCIDENTALLY took an Ambien (sleeping pill) instead of my antibiotic yesterday before I did an hour long training with a group of my agents! "Sorry Guys, this is going to be a short training. You've got 10 minutes to ask me questions." LOL. I totally crack myself up.

Would the wonderful person who ordered me Pizza Hut delivery last Friday please step forward?? It was great and it is driving me CRAZY that I don't know who did that for me.

I wanted to wish everyone a WONDERFUL HOLIDAY!! You are all the most amazing people in my life. I am so blessed! Thank you so much for all of the wonderful messages, phone calls, thoughts and prayers. Love you all, Connie

Wednesday, December 24, 2008 1:36 PM, CST

Connie, Stay strong girl! I know you can. You have many (sorority) sisters behind you sending their prayers. Including me! I hope you are able to have a great Holiday and can remember it through all your pain meds. :) I want you to know I am thinking of you and for a speedy recovery from this surgery. Hey PS —I work in Boro Park where everyone wears a wig, maybe I can get you a discount. I will check in frequently to see how you are doing. Judy G.

Thursday, December 25, 2008 5:36 PM, CST

If Santa is good to anyone we all know it will be you! Tried calling you tonight just to wish you a happy holiday since I knew you were with Mark. I laughed on the Ambien comment. I have my depilatory cream for my legs right next to my hairspray. Is that stupid or what. One of these days I am going to grab it by mistake, we both know that. Love you and hopefully you are getting some much needed rest.

Ellen

Friday, December 26, 2008 2:21 PM, CST

Hi Connie!!!

You continue to amaze me with your positive attitude and strength. I think you missed your calling in life! You should think about motivational speaking!!! You are a true inspiration to all!!! I got an email yesterday that said "When life hands you lemons, ask for tequila and salt and call me over!!!" It reminded me so much of you. I would love to come see you. Let me know when you are back in town. Happy New Year!!! xoxo Kristin D.

It is great to be with Mark and his family for Christmas. The house is buzzing with people and holiday spirit. I grew up with quiet holidays. Just my parents and my brother. Peaceful and quiet. I always wanted to experience the holidays as part of a big family. A happy family, unlike that of my ex-husband's, with its constant discord that became exhaustive and dreaded with each approaching holiday.

It is great for the most part, and hell for the other part. I was very reluctant to accompany Mark for the holidays for two reasons. One, because I always feel like I need a backup plan with him. I never feel like I can count on him for plans, and the more I look back on that very fact, the more idiotic I feel for having put up with it. And two, the traditional Italian Christmas Eve dinner consists solely of seafood (no pun intended) and I HATE seafood. It's a texture thing, a smell thing, and a taste thing. Trust me: it's just a thing, and not a good thing. So early on, I told Mark my fear of the dinner, not having anything to eat and looking like a moron because there might be no "normal" food for my consumption.

One of his aunts comes up to me and asks me why I'm not eating. I take Mark aside and tell him that there's nothing for me to eat. No "I'm sorry sweetie, let me get you something." He says, "Are you serious? I guess I can make you something." Come again? Did you not invite me here? Were you not aware that I was a fish-hater? Did you not assure me there would be other things for me to eat? I sit defeated in the room we share. This is the beginning of the Dr. Jekyll, Mr. Hyde #2 in my life. Another trip to Crazyville and I'm just not up for the journey. I realize, looking back on this evening, that his behavior was driven by alcohol and I made an excuse for it I guess. I needed to just get through.

He goes back out to his family to continue with the party while I sit in the room crying, thinking about grabbing my suitcase and driving home. Why am I even here? My brother is home for the holidays and I am here being treated like shit. I'm not having a pity party here, this is just a reality that I do not want to face. If I had possessed the physical and emotional fortitude, I would leave, drive the four hours home and never look back at Mark. Ever.

While there, my chest becomes huge and painful. Filled with fluid that has nowhere to drain. I actually wish that I have the drains back to relieve the pressure and the horrible pain. The only comparison that even comes close is to that of breast feeding. That feeling you have when your milk comes in. That tingle that tells you the baby needs to eat or you're going to explode. I breast-fed Alex, not Alyssa, and I think back to a time when my milk came in and he wasn't hungry. I had no pump, so I squeezed the milk out of my breast into a cup. I remember Derek coming into the room and saying, "What the hell are you doing?" I laugh at the thought, but unfortunately, there's no tingle this time, only pain. I spend the majority of the holiday icing my chest and loading up on Hydrocodone.

The thing that I need to mention here is that when you are married and your relationship is basically SHIT, you move on and find you are willing to put up with lesser or different versions of shit. Now that I am beyond this journey, I will tell you that I don't deal with ANY shit, but you do what you do to get through.

The rest of the holiday I spend walking on egg shells. I walk a wide berth around Mark. Careful not to set him off. I apologize (for what?) and do my best to deal. One thing I have learned, (and I think many women can relate to this) is that you do what you have to do to keep the peace. It's like that saying: Would you rather be happy, or would you rather be right? Personally, I'd rather be both. I mean, why not go for the whole enchilada?

We finally head home. Mark is all smiles and says, "We'll celebrate Christmas with the kids tomorrow night." He drops me off, and that is that. The next day comes and goes: no Mark. Again, we go through the "I ate some bad sushi" story I hear so often and the disappearing act starts again. Here's the thing. I am a very understanding person. Maybe it's the Scorpio in me that demands answers. I just want to know where I stand with people. And to constantly have to wonder where I stand with Mark is the most exhaustive process. A total mind-fuck: exhausting and never-ending. My marriage to Derek was a challenge in mental resilience, but at least with him, I knew what I was dealing with.

I remember thinking, "What am I doing? Why am I putting up with this shit?" I keep thinking, "Things will get better. When I am well, this relationship will be fun again." Hindsight is 20/20 as they say, and my hindsight is telling me that I should have cut my losses Christmas Day and bailed. We women are always questioning our "deserve" level when it comes to relationships. It has taken me half of my adult life to realize that I have a very high deserve level. A self-imposed "deserve" level that I will not sink beneath. I wish I had come to this revelation back then, but better late than never, right?

Tuesday, December 30, 2008 4:15 PM, CST

I hope all of you had a wonderful holiday! Mark and I had a great time down at his parents' house in Connecticut with all of his family. We celebrated Christmas with the kids when we got back, so we really had a good holiday.

I have been in a lot of pain for the last week since my drains were taken out. My plastic surgeon removed a lot of fluid from my chest this morning to relieve all of the pain and pressure I have been experiencing. Nothing a needle and a few Percocets can't cure!

So I had the much dreaded oncology appointment today. I am in good spirits, but seriously, how much information can one person digest in a day? I am having a heart scan on Friday, a bone scan and CAT scan next Wednesday and then my lymph node surgery next Friday along with the Mediport implant for chemo. So the chemo situation is this—8 treatments, once every 2 weeks. So 16 weeks, and it will all be over! My cancer is estrogen-driven, so I will have to be on hormone therapy for 5 years after I complete my treatments. And yes, I am going to lose my hair. On the bright side, I won't have to pluck my eyebrows for awhile or shave. That's a plus, right?

Everyone keeps asking me, what do you need? What can I do? I SO APPRECIATE all of you, your thoughts and prayers, cards and phone calls. You all know that I'd rather do everything myself because that's just how I am. BUT, I am realizing now that I can't. The smallest of tasks makes me tired and I am used to running at 100 mph. So I am going to ask you all for help. I know that I am going to need help getting to appointments, help when I feel like CRAP after treatments and help with the kids. And I definitely know that I will not be feeling up to being Rachael Ray while I go through this, so all of your offers of dinners I will take with much appreciation!

I will get through this with a sense of humor and come out of it with the same sense of humor (hopefully).

I hope all is well with everyone! Happy New Year! And thank you so much for all of the great messages!

Love, Connie :)

Tuesday, December 30, 2008 6:48 PM, CST

Hi Connie,

Just a note from New Jersey to say that we have been reading your updates as soon as they are written and we are thinking about you constantly. The coming New Year brings with it lots of reflection and no one is more on our minds or in our hearts than you, Alex and Alyssa. Though the situation is scary and overwhelming, having a plan is empowering. Here's to new beginnings and to restored health in 2009. Love, Jon, Mindy & Quincy R.

Tuesday, December 30, 2008 7:14 PM, CST

Connie,

My word, girlfriend, you are an inspiration to all. We are supposed to be inspiring you and look at you...inspiring everyone else. You do amaze me.

Here is a quote from Mark Twain

"Courage is resistance to fear, mastery of fear—not absence of fear."

You are courageous, and you are ready to fight that fear... and you can do it and beat it. Not a day goes by that I don't think of you...God Bless you and yours...LOVE Nancy D.

Tuesday, December 30, 2008 8:20 PM, CST

Connie, It is that sense of humor that you have which will pull you through the toughest times. Stay strong. I wish I lived closer to offer kid pick up, food cooking, but I don't. All I can offer are my prayers and good wishes. If you ever need to talk just pick up the phone. Keep the faith and take one day at a time. Love ya, Judy G.

Tuesday, December 30, 2008 11:22 PM, CST

Connie,

I am just reading my emails from all of December! Michelle emailed me about your site, and I'm so glad I logged on. She also told me of all the impending tests and surgeries. Yuck!! Next week will be THE WEEK to PRAY< PRAY< PRAY for you. Just telling you again that you are in my heart and mind constantly. Every time you feel down, remember that I am here holding you up in prayer and holding you TIGHT in LOVE, wherever you are, no matter what is happening…and I won't let go of you, ever! You are so special to us. I don't know when it is a good time to call, and your week looks pretty filled up! So call me so we can talk. I want to help!! Lots of love and hugs,

Mrs. G. (Laura)

Wednesday, December 31, 2008 7:52 AM, CST

Hey there you…wow just a little shit to deal with huh???? I am off on Tuesdays so if you want/need rides or just someone to bring lunch and bull shit or clean the house… Lets plan for it OK…Keeping you in my prayers…Love ya girl…Laura D.

Wednesday, December 31, 2008 9:14 AM, CST

Connie! I am laughing mixed in with my tears while reading your entry. Aren't we supposed to make you laugh? My heart goes out to you and your family. When I read your words of course I hear your voice and I think to myself this girl is going to make it through this and be better than she was before. You are an inspiration to all of us and I can't imagine how many people you will help in your lifetime because of this journey. I hope you received the pictures I sent you. That was one of the funniest weekends ever in Mary Kay. I couldn't resist the ones with the hairpieces specifically. I can't wait to see you in January. If I get to cast my vote…I say pink. Love you and miss you.

Joan F.

Chapter 7
Dr. Death and Friends

The day I meet my oncologist, Dr. L, I know immediately that I will like him. He is young, attractive and has a great sense of humor. Mark takes me to the appointment. It is an informative meeting. It amazes me how these doctors can be so matter-of-fact with your odds of survival. Percentages and graphs are laid before me. I stare at them, not really hearing that I have a 70 percent chance of survival after five years if I do this, 80 percent chance if I do that. My vision is blurred by the tears that have come to my eyes after hearing I will not be able to have any more children. That my cancer is estrogen-driven and, therefore, carrying another child is not an option. It's one thing to make the choice of your own volition, another to have it made for you. Especially given the fact that Mark has no children of his own and I thought at some point we would have one together. Dr. L gives us a few minutes alone and I sob. The first time I have cried in weeks. I look to Mark and cry, "I'm so sorry. I understand if you don't want to be with me because of this." Again, with the "deserve" level!

Looking back on that moment, I realize that was MY issue, not his. Again with my thoughts of the fairy tale, the happy ending. If there is one thing that I have taken away from this life-changing experience, it is that I need to put myself first. That no man in my life is worth shelving myself, even for a moment, in order to meet a mold I think I should fit for them. The realization that he didn't even care about having a child with me, makes me feel foolish. Here I am receiving my life sentence, all the while worrying that I can't give a man I loved dearly a child.

New Year's comes and goes. The kids, Mark and I spend a lazy New Year's together. It is nice. I bought Mark the first season of *House* on DVD for Christmas, so we watched episode after episode, relaxed, ate good food and ushered in the new year. It is peaceful. It is the calm before the storm. Will I be able to keep my ship upright? My kids, my skipper and first mate. I need to keep this ship sailing for them even through the toughest of storms. My ship has survived a stormy divorce; is it strong enough to withstand the rocky waters and high winds of an illness? I was about to find out.

The time comes for me to tell my kids I have breast cancer. I remember as a child, my parents taking me to the drive-in theater. The speaker hung on the drivers' door, the window wide open letting in a mass of mosquitoes as my parents and I sat watching Bambi. I was five or six years old, but I remember it like it was yesterday. A hunter's rifle blasts and Bambi's mother lay dead in the woods. As Bambi hovered over her dead mother, I cried and was completely inconsolable for the remainder of the movie. I remember this feeling of tremendous sadness. I think it was the first time in my life that I understood what loss was. When my mother was diagnosed with breast cancer, I sat in the hospital waiting room thinking of Bambi. How would I live without my mother?

Years later, when my mother was buried, I sat at her gravesite thinking of that movie. Sitting on my mother's lap, watching the fate of a little doe on a larger-than-life screen. It's funny how memories from your childhood burn into the core of your being. Now I had grown from a lost little doe to a mother. My greatest fear was to have my kids hover over me dead in the woods.

I was so tormented at the thought of having this conversation with them. How do you tell two little kids that their mom has breast cancer? That she will probably be sick for months and will most definitely be bald?

I take a deep breath and ask them to sit with me on the couch. Debra gave me a children's book to help me explain it. I start to read the book called *The Paper Chain*. I am grateful for the visual aid. The power of the pictures for the kids, the power of words for me.

The book mentions cancer and Alyssa looks at me and says, "Mom, do you have cancer?" I say yes and that I will be OK. I tell them that I have breast cancer and that I need to have chemotherapy like the Mommy in the book. I will be bald and we will have fun picking out wigs. Alyssa immediately makes the connection to my mother's death and has a meltdown. I've always told my children the truth. Now I feel as if I have to lie about my health in order to protect them.

And so I do.

I try not to cry as I tell them what lies ahead. All the while I think, "I will be fine. I will be fine." Do I know this for sure? Hell no!

The kids seem OK after our chat. My little Alex says, "Mom, it's not like you're going to die or something."

I nod my head and say, "You're absolutely right." At least HE'S confident. "Well, little man," I think, "I hope you are right."

The conversation ends with Alex wanting me to get a green-haired wig; Alyssa wants a pink one. We will have fun with this, even if it kills me.

No pun intended.

I appeal to the masses for help with my wig selection. A voting frenzy ensues

Tuesday, January 6, 2009 4:03 PM, CST

So I need help with something. I am on a hunt for a wig, as I don't want to seem totally freakish as a bald woman. I am imagining myself looking like one of those bald vampire people in *I Am Legend* with Will Smith. If you haven't seen it, watch it and you will laugh thinking of me looking like one of them.

So here's the scoop. I need all of you (when you have any spare time) to go onto www.wigs.com and take a look. I have two that I like, but there are SO MANY. So one I like is the Revlon "Scorpio" wig, which is ironic because I am a Scorpio. What a laugh! The other one is the John Renau "Posh" wig, which would be like my old "do" before the recent "chop off" which I can't stand. So please look and let me know if either one is good or if there is another one that would look alright. I already know Alyssa is going to vote for the pink one on the site. Alex will probably pick the one that has green in it. NOT GOING TO HAPPEN.

So I told the kids last night that I have breast cancer. Alex was fine. He's seven. He thinks I'm the "best Mom ever." Yeah, that's going to last forever! LOL. So he was OK. Alyssa on the other hand, at eight knows how my mother passed away from breast cancer and had a total freak attack. She is OK now. They both know that I am going to lose my hair and we are going to have a blast with the wigs. Now they both want their own. Go figure!

Well, take a look at the website and let me know what you guys think!!

Love ya!

Con:)

Tuesday, January 6, 2009 3:28 PM, CST

Girlfriend, I have to go for the Scorpio. LOVE the pink highlights. Hugs and smiles. You're the bomb. —Kathryn G.

Tuesday, January 6, 2009 3:44 PM, CST

Connie,

I will go take a look, but I just wanted to say that I think you are amazing.

Wendy C.

Tuesday, January 6, 2009 4:02 PM, CST

Connie,

I totally vote for the posh. It's perfect!

Keep fighting the fight.

Love,

Linda Z.

Tuesday, January 6, 2009 4:42 PM, CST

LOVE THE POSH!

Joan F.

Tuesday, January 6, 2009 5:59 PM, CST

Connnstaaannnce! I am lovin the posh

Dude I do the breast cancer run every year...(I know you can't picture my arse runnin) but I do and I can't wait to do it in honor of you next October chick I love ya!!! :)

Andrea G.

Chapter 8
Wig and Treasure Hunts

*T*he thought of wearing a wig is daunting. Throwing a rug on my head every day is not the most appealing thought, but the alternative seems much worse. I use the wig hunt as an excuse to get my kids involved in the process. With a seven year old and an eight year old, I not only have to think of my own sanity, but their sanity as well. Turning cancer into an "adventure" seems to be my only plan.

When I was a kid, we lived near a campsite. Almost daily, my brother and I would ride our bikes at the site, meandering down all of the streets and perusing the lots. Never in a million years would I allow my children to do that. We even rode bikes without helmets, and somehow we are alive to tell about it. My, how things have changed. I remember days when our Mom would come with us and say, "Kids, let's go exploring." The three of us would pretend to be on some sort of an adventure, seeking out unknowns of the world—flat rocks that we could skip across the lake or acorns with crazy-shaped tops. My kids are not going to be experiencing the freeness of that type of exploration. At least not now. How can I bring them into the fold of something as dark as cancer and make it "light?"

As I formulated in my head days earlier how I would tell them, I realized that in order for all of us to survive this, it was up to me to make it an adventure. The wig became the adventure. It became a family affair. Alyssa wanted a pink wig, Alex a green one. When I told them I would still be coming to school for their events and actually be WEARING the wig, they decided that a crazy-colored wig would not be in their best interest.

My mind switches gears to my next upcoming surgery. It is three days away, and I am getting nervous. The removal of a bunch of lymph nodes in my arm and the insertion of a Mediport for chemo. When I tell my ex-husband that he will need to take the kids again for a couple of days for this surgery, he responds with, "Well, you know ah, you can ah, take chemo by a pill now ya know."

To which I respond with, "Well Derek, my oncologist has decided my best chances for survival are to crush up the pills, mix them with water and insert them through a needle into the port they will put in my chest." WTF! Don't you think that if I could swallow a freaking PILL, I would? How ever did I do it, I wonder.

Thursday, January 8, 2009 3:57 PM, CST

How cool it has been to hear from all of you! Especially my Sorority Sisters!! What intoxicating times those were!! Plattsburgh State didn't know what hit it! LOL!

So I didn't have my CAT and bone scans yesterday because school was closed due to the weather and Alex was sick (still is) with the stomach bug. I hope I don't get it until after my surgery!

I am a little nervous about tomorrow. I'm not too psyched about going under the knife again. Now I know exactly what my mother meant about being a human pin cushion. I had fluid drained from my chest again today, but my plastic surgeon said everything looks great and that the fluid buildup happens to some of his patients. Tomorrow I will be getting the dreaded drains back in. Mark gave me a fanny pack to put them in so they don't just hang (which is painful). Last time I had the drains, that fanny pack drove me CRAZY because every time I walked I could hear myself coming and going with the rattle of the zippers!! Now when I walk, I just hear the slosh of fluid in my "almost boobs." Have to find humor somewhere :)

So my plastic surgeon told me today that my ETA for new boobs will be sometime this summer. 2–3 weeks after my last chemo treatment, when my white blood cell count is high enough, I can get my new "girls" with yet ANOTHER surgery. At least one part of me won't be sagging when my kids slap me into a home.

I hope all of you are well. Thanks so much for the great messages! The kids and I have been surfing the net for wigs and I will go to a salon and get fitted for one (thank you Dotte C for looking into all of that for me!!). Alyssa wants me to be "funky." Am I not already??

I will see how drugged up I am tomorrow after my surgery and let you all know how I made out. If my writing is slurred, then you will know I'm on some good stuff!!

Love to all! Con :)

Thursday, January 8, 2009 7:49 PM, CST

Connie, you wonderful woman you, I'm so sorry to hear about all you're dealing with. My thoughts and prayers are with you. Hang in there—I have no doubt that with your strength you have what it takes to get through this. I love you and will be pulling for you all the way! This cancer should be very afraid—it has no idea the strength of an AD! :) Love, hugs and kisses Con!

Julie C.

Thursday, January 8, 2009 10:05 PM, CST

Connie, OK are you allowed to curse on this thing or will everybody get upset. I can't go without calling you at least an ass or a douche bag...for old time's sake anyway. Let's make a deal...give me the name of the doctor who gives you a pair of new boobs (you know I wanted to put something else in there), and see if he can get me a new twat (cervical cancer). We can do this kid...I'm right here for you...always. When you're up to it, drop me a line so I can come up and help you out or curse at you, or teach your kids some bad stuff, or curse at your boyfriend...or just hold your hand. Seriously, without the vulgarity...I love you and miss you and want to be there for you through this. All my love to you, and my prayers to you and your family.

Ginny R.

OMG!! Note to self, tell Ginny that my Dad reads my journal and everyone's entries!!

Friday, January 9, 2009 9:15 AM, CST

You're in my thoughts and prayers! I love you, Connie... hugs, Ellen D.

Chapter 9
Port of Call

The day of my next surgery arrives. My friend Amy accompanies Mark and me to the procedure. It is a long day that starts with having ink inserted into the lymph nodes in my arm to see which ones to remove. Amy and Mark kept each other entertained as I lie there drugged and waiting for my surgery to begin. My surgery keeps getting delayed because of another patient's surgery. Later I will find out it was a girl I knew from high school who trumped my surgery. She and I along on this same journey together.

No one can ever accuse me of not having a sense of humor. After my surgeon marks me up for surgery, he makes the mistake of leaving the semi-permanent marker on the table in my room. And in my happy juiced state, I allow Mark and Amy to write on my belly with said ink. I get wheeled into the operating room, and as they transfer me from the bed to the operating table, my gown opens and reveals, "We love Dr. B" on my abdomen. I fall asleep to sounds of uproarious laughter.

I wake up as I am being rolled back to my room for a quick recovery before being discharged, all the while hearing laughter from the operating room nurses at my friends' latest attempt at graffiti. I get back to my room where my rebellious artist friends await me. A nurse asks me if she can get me anything to drink and I respond with, "Yes, a Cosmopolitan." No doubt, I desperately need one, especially if I had the foresight to know it will take TWO WEEKS to get the writing off my stomach!

Saturday, January 10, 2009 12:23 PM, CST

Hi Everybody!! I survived my surgery yesterday!! It was pushed back 4 hours due to an emergency surgery, but they kept giving IV pushes of what I fondly call "whoohoo" to keep me calm and "happy." Mark and my friend Amy are new BFF's from spending so much time together yesterday waiting for my surgery. My surgeon Dr. B marked me up with a permanent marker for surgery and made the mistake of leaving the marker on my table. Mark and Amy thought it would be funny to write a message on my body for my surgeon. So they wrote "We love Dr. B" on my abdomen while I was full of "whoohoo." Apparently, it was great entertainment for the entire surgical staff, and now I have a semi-permanent reminder of the message.

I had a blue dye injection in my arm (which has left a really ugly "tattoo" that looks like I've been beaten) to see where there was any cancer. I was a bit loopy when Dr. B talked to me, but he removed A LOT of lymph nodes. I think he said 20. The surgery was 2 1/2 hrs long. Dr. B said that he had to split one of my nerves to get at a spot, so I will not get feeling back on one part of my arm. This whole process has split more than one of my nerves, trust me!

He placed the Mediport for chemo on my right side above my breast area (or my NON-breast area right now). It is very strange to have something protruding from under your skin. My first thought was "when is this thing going to come out?" I'm stuck with it for a few months I guess.

I'm a little surprised at my pain level. Thank goodness for Lortab! My left arm is very sore and I have very limited range of motion. Blow drying my hair this morning was a real challenge. Good thing I chopped it all off. I'm one chop away from Sinead O'Connor. Need to take baby steps to baldness!

Amy stayed overnight with me last night for a post surgical "girls night." So I go to the bathroom last night and my pee is green! I yell, "Aim, my pee is green!" We are geniuses because we figured out that yellow (pee) and blue (dye) = GREEN. We were so proud of ourselves!! What a laugh!! It might have been helpful if we had been given a "heads up" about the green pee.

I am doing well, especially with Lortab. Thanks so much for all of your messages!!

Love, Con :)

Saturday, January 10, 2009 8:35 AM, CST

Connie,

Thinking of you/sending prayers your way.

Pam H.

Saturday, January 10, 2009 12:13 PM, CST

Care to share the drugs...????? LOL I am so impressed with your emails and attitude towards everything... I really hope it's not a front so that we are all sitting here reading your ever-so-positive emails and you are sitting there with your head hung low. Knowing you as little as I do, you need to be Miss Mary Sunshine to all...Anyway, I am so, so glad that things went well yesterday...hopefully the kids are doing well with all of this. Hey listen regarding the hair, I cut mine mega mega short like, need to get it cut every three weeks no longer, and let it go completely gray. So the next time you see me need your honest thoughts...Take it easy enjoy the drugs while you can but don't enjoy them too much don't want to have to put you on that show in TV intervention...lol take care my best and Jim sends his Prayers to you...Laura D

Saturday, January 10, 2009 12:58 PM, CST

Connie—Just wanted you to know I'm thinking of you—and I'm glad everything went OK yesterday. All my love—Jules

Saturday, January 10, 2009 4:24 PM, CST

Hi Connie,

I've been thinking about you today and wish I were closer to give you a hug, so you will have to accept the virtual one until I get up there this summer. I read how brave you are for your children and want to let you know you can call me anytime if you need to talk. Let me know when you are up to a call.

Love you lots

Cindy B.

Saturday, January 10, 2009 9:19 PM, CST

Connie, One more major hurdle over with. I thought and prayed for you yesterday. About the green pee...Blue dye does that. Just let your kids eat a couple of blue airheads and that's what occurs when they go poop. LOL. Keep strong. I agree with Margaret purple wigs for Homecoming!!!!!!!!!

Was the marker purple too?? Next step chemo…one more major hurdle to get over with. If you need anything just call. Thinking of you every day. Love, Judy G.

Saturday, January 10, 2009 10:54 PM, CST

Gotta love those surgeons Connie. The Mediport is the greatest thing…I know it feels uncomfortable right now, but it will save you from needle sticks for blood draws and chemo. This way, you won't get the "chemo veins." Let's give Julie M. a call and see if she can give you some of her mane. We'll get you whipped up into one of those 80's do's in a snap. Keep your head up chicky…thinking of you all the time, praying for you all the time, and sending my love to you all the time. Ginny R.

Sunday, January 11, 2009 10:29 AM, CST

I read your entries and I laugh and cry at the same time. Your wit on this entire procedure is done with elegance and grace and that huge dose of humor that all of us know and love about you. You should write something every day and for any of the entries you've included here, you should make sure to cut and paste them to your journal including the dates. The Memoirs of "Connie…us" could make for a great read, I know (and can hear) how hard you are laughing and hopefully you're the only one that gets it!

So you are home already? God, modern medicine might be advancing way too quickly as it would seem a day or two to have someone look after you would be a huge help.

Again, Connie, I am thinking of you and just want you to know that. I will call you tomorrow. I love you! xoxo Ellen D.

Sunday, January 11, 2009 5:13 PM, CST

> Well hello, Miss Connie!!! You are a hoot!!! So glad your spirits are good. A positive attitude makes all the difference. Glad your surgery went well. You are in my thoughts and prayers every day. Take care.
>
> Debbie D.

I need to take a moment to tell you about the port in my chest. It pretty much sucks. I'm grateful that I will not have to endure the prodding and probing of needles in my arm for all of my chemo treatments, but in keeping it real, having a foreign object implanted in your chest is not in the least bit pleasant. I lie there the night of the surgery, running my fingers over the hexagonal object embedded in my chest. I wonder if it has a tracking device. I can just see my oncologist looking at my location. "Nurse, we need an intervention! She's at Macy's!" Either that, or at the nearest pub, choking down copious amount of alcohol to help me forget about the port in my chest. I wonder if I can have an intravenous line of vodka straight through the port, so as to save me the physical exertion of drinking. I assume at some point, all activity will be nothing short of exhausting.

Having cancer is almost a "dirty" feeling. The immediate reaction is to rid yourself of the dirt by bathing, akin to falling into a puddle of mud. Instead of looking at the dirt on your arm and thinking, "I need to take a bath," you think about something dirty that is invisible to the naked eye, something that is running through your veins that you can't get rid of. It's always there even when you can't see it. At least the thought of it anyway.

I think back to a moment in my married life. I got up early one morning to iron my clothes for work and as I was ironing, my husband slept. Not getting the kids up and ready for daycare, but sleeping. I remember thinking, "I wonder if I could kill him with this iron and make it look like a shaving accident." My mind then reels to "the scene," homicide detectives looking over the body, looking for cause of death, motive. Undoubtedly, the steam holes from the iron would leave a mark on his face and blow my whole story. I contemplate the eradication of my cancer. The chemotherapy I am about to endure is going to leave hole marks from the iron, not a nick from a razor. The thought of becoming bald looms closer.

Monday, January 12, 2009 7:08 AM, CST

I am a bit cranky. The pain from this surgery has really thrown me for a loop. I am in great spirits, but extremely tired from lack of sleep because there is NO comfortable position to sleep in. I have lost A LOT of feeling in my left arm that is permanent from the surgery. I have no feeling on the back side of my arm from the shoulder down to my elbow. It is very strange. I know I will get through this, but the pain is just getting on my nerves because it is hard to move around. Trying to move around reminds of the girl in the body brace from *"Sixteen Candles."* It will get better I know.

Does anyone know of any organizations that foster animals for a period of time? I am having a hard time taking care of Abe, our 90 pound chocolate lab. He is 11 years old. I was hoping to find a temporary home for him until I complete my chemo because I am having a hard enough time keeping up with the kids, let alone the dog and I know it will get tougher. He is a great dog, and I don't want to give him up for adoption because I know the kids will be crushed. So if anyone knows of any organizations that could help, please let me know. I am going to call my vet today and ask her.

This afternoon I have my next oncology appointment to set up my schedule for chemo and have the doctor explain it to me a little more in detail. My friend Missy mentioned to me how I can have an online calendar with all of my appointments so that everyone knows when I need help. Once I find out the schedule, I am going to try to get that all figured out so I know that I have rides to all of my appointments. Thanks to all of you who have offered to take me. I really appreciate it.

Will keep you all posted on this afternoon.

Love, Connie

Monday, January 12, 2009 4:42 PM, CST

Hang in there Connie. You are entitled to be cranky every once and a while and more often than not is OK. You just need to take care of yourself! Love ya, Cindy B.

Monday, January 12, 2009 6:00 PM, CST

Connie—so glad that the surgery went well…Keep up that positive attitude!!!!!!!!!!!! I am keeping you in my prayers…Love ya, Liz M.

Tuesday, January 13, 2009 1:41 AM, CST

Hello Connie!

Sending Hugs and Kisses to you, Alyssa, and Alex :) :) :)

Love,

Gina P.

Tuesday, January 13, 2009 7:12 AM, CST

Hey Con…so sorry to hear you are in a lot of "discomfort," as we call it in the med field (we try not to use pain) as it psyches you out of it or something…I didn't call you back because I had forgotten you were back in the hospital for more surgery so I figured it wasn't a good time. You just call me when you can. Also, I have a good friend Amy who is a foster dog mom!!! How wild. I will call you with her number right away. I think there is a process for her group but she can certainly point you in the right direction if she can't care for Abe herself...I love you sweetie. Get rest. Get better.

Jen K.

Tuesday, January 13, 2009 9:53 AM, CST

Connie,

Keep your chin up. You'll get through this. And you are entitled to be cranky! I can probably babysit your dog for a while. I love chocolate labs. Call me!

Elena T.

Chapter 10
Superheros and Villains

I believe I am Superwoman. The mom who does everything; the woman who does everything. Most importantly, the caregiver who can continue to give care, even though I am not at my 100 percent running speed. My surgeon gave me a heads up that I would have limited arm mobility, but again, I think I'm Superwoman, so I can handle it. Having cancer has made me realize and ACCEPT that I have limitations. Caring for Abe became unbearably painful. Physically, it was a challenge just to hold him to put him on his runner. And mentally, I had this constant argument with myself about my ability to care for him. It was fine when the kids were home because they helped me, but when they were with their dad, I was all alone and it became difficult. After much contemplation, I had to choose myself over Abe.

Thursday, January 15, 2009 8:14 AM, CST

> I had to go to my surgeon's office yesterday because my chest drain has been leaking. My pathology results were in and I HAVE NO POSITIVE LYMPH NODES!! The news could not be better!! Now I definitely won't need radiation! I am so happy and so RELIEVED! My prognosis has been good all along, but now it is even better!

Now I just have to get through these 8 chemo treatments and deal with hormone therapy for 5 years (which I am still on the fence about) and I will be around for a LONG TIME!

I got home and told the kids the good news. They were so happy (of course) but still don't understand why I have to have the "treatments" since the cancer is gone. I told them I am having the treatments so that I can be their Mom for a long time. Alex said, "Mom, you're the best mom ever." Thank Goodness!

So I am still trying to figure out the best scenario for Abe. He pulled on my arm yesterday when I was letting him out and it just about killed me. I really need to have him be in better care while I get healthy. I need to get him situated within the next week or so.

I am definitely feeling better. The pain from this surgery has really shocked me. Nothing a heating pad and a few Hydrocodones can't fix!

When I am feeling better, I need to get situated with a wig. My insurance company may cover the cost so I am going to check into that today before I make any appointments for fittings. I would love to go with a bunch of girlfriends and make it a day. I will need lots of laughs to get through this one!

I am having my CAT scan and bone scan tomorrow. My friend Lisa is taking me, so I know we will definitely be laughing through the whole thing. Now that my lymph nodes are clear, I won't be too stressed about the outcome of these scans.

I hope this note finds everyone well and WARM even though we are going through a "deep freeze." I can't believe how cold it is!

Love to all, Connie :)

Thursday, January 15, 2009 9:17 AM, CST

FANFREAKENTASIC NEWS!!!!! How awesome is that I am so happy for you!!!! I also could hear Alex saying, "you're the best mom" haha so damn cute.

I love ya girl ! We will talk soon ;)

Andrea G.

Thursday, January 15, 2009 9:22 AM, CST

Oh Con, I'm SOOO happy and relieved for you. What wonderful news. I know it's still a struggle but what a hurdle you must feel you've jumped! You call me if you want to do a girls thing for the wigs—we've moved but my cell is the same—I'll try calling you this weekend. I love you and am praying for you every day! You're never out of my thoughts—hang in there! Jules

Thursday, January 15, 2009 9:50 AM, CST

THE TEARS ARE STREAMING DOWN MY FACE WITH JOY!!!!!!!!!!!!! MY SISTER FROM ANOTHER MOTHER I LOVE YOU AND PRAY FOR YOUR PEACEFUL JOURNEY. LOOK OUT TATTOO PARLOR HERE WE COME! PERHAPS ONE ON YOUR TUSH THAT SAYS "CANCER—YOU CAN KISS MY A@#!!!!"

XOXOXOXOXOXOXOXOXOXO TO YOU AND THE BABES.

Laurie K.

Thursday, January 15, 2009 10:36 AM, CST

Connie...I am so happy for you. What an amazing update! You are back in control and I am sure (knowing what I know about you) you are feeling lots of relief. It was so so so good to finally talk to you and I am looking forward to seeing you next Friday.

Joan F.

The news of not needing any radiation is a godsend. I have finally caught a break. I remember my brother and I taking turns taking our mother for radiation when she was undergoing her breast cancer treatment. Her face always wore the signs of being so tired, even though she put on such a brave face for the rest of us. I knew it wore on her and I felt a bit selfish at my relief. I wish I could say to her, "Mom, I know how you must have felt." Instead, I look up to the sky as I leave my surgeon's office, telling myself I have made it through one hurdle and have many more to jump over. I'm just hoping I can get over these hurdles, unlike the ones I unsuccessfully would jump over in gym class as a kid. I imagine myself face-first on the track, gravel embedded in my knees as I refuse to lose this next track meet.

Chapter 11
Marcus Welby, MD

I n the days following my surgery, I have a CAT scan and a MUGGA scan. For the CAT scan I have to drink this horrible chalky stuff that makes me gag. I'm a chick who doesn't eat seafood because of texture and would be the first person to write my name down on the parchment on *Survivor* for having to eat something not found on the menu of an All-American restaurant. So imagine me gagging every fifteen minutes for two hours as I choke down the chalky beverage. Here I am, a woman who has basically had her breasts lobbed off and I am having issues with a chalky beverage. Go figure.

The CAT scan is performed to view my entire body for the spread of cancer. The MUGGA scan is used to give a baseline as to my heart function because the chemotherapy I will be receiving can affect heart function. I survive them both. More pokes and prods with needles. I'd better get used to it, because this is only the beginning.

Friday, January 16, 2009 3:54 PM, EST

I swear Alan Funt (sp?) from *Candid Camera* is lurking somewhere in my house at all times watching all of my antics.

"Smile, you're on *Candid Camera*!" It has been that kind of week.

I think I wrote about the problem with my chest drain leaking. It's like a *Seinfeld* episode. It was leaking from my chest (not through the tube) on Tuesday night, so I went to see my surgeon on Wednesday and that's when I got my great news. Well, he tried to get the fluid to flow through the tube and we thought all was a success so I went on my merry way.

Wednesday night it leaked ALL NIGHT LONG, had to change my clothes, blah, blah. I have to wear this ridiculous "surgical bra" at all times that is oh so attractive, and I only have 3. I was up doing laundry all night. So yesterday morning I'm thinking I'm Dr. Marcus Welby and I'm going to fix it once and for all. Long story short, THE ENTIRE TUBE CAME OUT OF MY CHEST AND FELL OUT ON THE FLOOR! "Smile, you're on *Candid Camera*!" Unbelievable! Not to gross anyone out, but there was about 6–8 inches of tubing that was INSIDE my chest cavity. Oh, and I found the reason for the blockage—a clot that looked like an earthworm! Mark was in Buffalo so I called him to tell him and he said, "You'd better save it and bring it in to the doctor's." Well, that's attractive. Of course I did, and my doctor laughed. He's still laughing over the "We love Dr. B" note on my stomach from my recent surgery.I have to thank my friend Lisa H. who is a total sport for taking me to the doctor's yesterday and also today for taking me for my scans. We got to the doctor's yesterday and the nurse says, "Here comes trouble." And of course my dear friend has to add, "You have NO idea!" We had lots of laughs.

I had my CAT scan and bone scan today. Before I got there, I had to force myself to drink that horrible stuff. UGH!

Honestly, it just about killed me. I know, I have issues! I would never make it on "*Survivor.*" I'd be the first one to vote myself off!

The guy who injected me for my CAT scan said, "Now I am going to inject the contrast. It is going to give you a warm sensation in the back of your throat and it will work its way down to your pelvis and you will feel like you are peeing your pants, but you really aren't peeing your pants." To which I respond with "Bonus!" I felt like Jodie Foster in *Contact* with the hoopy thing circling around me like it did her on her way to that planet. So many parallels, LOL! This whole thing is such an adventure. Lisa, thanks for all the laughs today and yesterday!!

I want to thank Dotte C. and her daughter Trish for help with placing Abe while I get well. You are such AMAZING women to help me! Trish has a friend who is a veterinarian who has offered to help me with Abe and I am truly grateful. I can't imagine him being in better care. I will be taking him to her tomorrow.

Thank you all for the notes, well wishes and laughs! I am doing great! The pain is still there with my arm, but it can only get better. I start my chemo on February 11th and if everything goes according to plan, I will have my last treatment on May 20th. I can live through anything for 4 months!

I hope this note finds all of you well. Thanks again for being such wonderful friends to me!!

Love, Connie :)

Friday, January 16, 2009 3:35 PM, CST

OK ff...my last note got lost, so if you didn't get it, I hope you remember what ff means...hint...it starts with an "F", and ends with "Face." I think God has been listening to all of us...thank you God for the great news! Connie, just to let you know, I have an incredible amount of knowledge when it comes to chemo and all the rest of it, so if there's something you forget to talk to your doctor about or you just want to talk, please call me. Drop me a note if you have time on email so I can send a curse-filled greeting to you! Have a little celebration this weekend with your man and kids, and make sure you do something good for you...like a pedi/mani...I can't do that for myself because when the Chinese ladies see me in the parking lot, they close the shop for the day...my toes are like bamboo sticks...ha ha. Love ya girl... keep smiling,

Ginny R.

OMG! I am going to KILL her!

Friday, January 16, 2009 4:19 PM, CST

Hey Connie,

It sounds like things are going well for you. I am so happy to hear that the test came back with happy news! I have my whole family praying for ya.

Soccer has been brutal. We went from first to last in a matter of seconds it seems. Getting bruised and battered— but as sadistic as I am, I love it, it's too much fun. The ladies on the team were asking for ya, so when you feel up to it, please come by for a visit, we could use a cheering section!

I am up for the wig party, so keep me in mind, I would love to hang with ya and get you looking hot in your new "do." Have you thought about big curly 80's hair, you know kinda like mine— at least that is what Eryn calls it (as if she knows anything about the 80's!). Well anyway, it's been fun for me (wink wink).

I am really happy that the news I keep hearing is good— keep strong and keep smiling!

Love ya—

Jen B.

Friday, January 16, 2009 4:42 PM, CST

Dear Connie,

Thanks for taking the time to write your updates. I read them all and isn't it great to have your friends helping you out in any and all ways?!:) You are a courageous woman— live one day at a time and keep your sense of humor. You are amazing!!! We love you Connie. Maureen and Gene L.

Friday, January 16, 2009 5:22 PM, CST

Lady…you are just too funny. You will be able to write a book when this is all over. Keep notes of your adventures. It will be a bestseller Connie, I haven't heard from you regarding helping you with the dog on Saturday. My earlier message was I would meet you at your house if you need help getting him in the car or I can meet you at the vet's office so I can hold the leash and you won't run the risk of getting hurt. The vet might be busy and we would have to wait a bit. I can help you with Abe's "stuff" so you won't

have to carry it. Call me and we can make a plan to get Abe
squared away tomorrow.

Dotte C.

It completely amazes me how so many people can come to your rescue
when you are at a low point in your life. My friends are wonderful, rallying
to find a place for Abe for awhile so I can deal with my illness. My ex finally
came through for me and found someone who would take Abe for a couple of
weeks while I healed. I missed having him around to keep me company, but I
definitely did not miss the tumbleweeds of dog hair that would appear out of
thin air.

The whole "drain falling out of my chest" mess was quite a calamity. The
tube mysteriously became unstitched from my skin. OK, I might have cut it
with scissors, but I wasn't expecting the whole tube to come flying out of my
body while I was in the shower! A dozen flies could have flown in my mouth
while I stood there agape at the comedy that was literally unraveling from me. I
contemplated stuffing the tube back in and pretending the stitches came loose,
but when I looked at the actual length of the tube, I said "Screw it! I'll just tell
my surgeon it fell out in the shower. Maybe he'll buy my story."

I call the surgeon's office and inform them of the tube incident. They ask
me to come up as soon as possible so they can assess the damage. The nurse
informs me that the doctor may have to reinsert the drain in his office. Are you
shitting me? Seriously?

I get to the surgeon's office, and the nurse says to Lisa and I, "It's a bit nipply
out there isn't it?" Probably not the best way to express extreme cold to a patient
who just had her nipples removed along with her breasts, but hey, what are ya
gonna do?

I tell her, "Well actually, my nipple thermometer is no longer in working
order." I am kidding, but I think she searches for the nearest jaws of life to
extricate her foot from her mouth. The doctor comes in, examines my drainage
site, and to my immediate relief, decides not to reinsert a new drain. Another
bullet dodged.

The poking and prodding continues and I basically feel as if I LIVE at the local hospital, surgeon's office and oncologist's office. I contemplate backpacking to each appointment and pitching a tent.

Why not? I'll be here tomorrow anyways!

Tuesday, January 20, 2009 6:35 PM, CST

The adventure continues. Today my friend Rene (You're the best Rene) took me to my two surgical appointments. First stop, drain the breasts. So I had 100 cc's of fluid removed from my left side and I feel SO MUCH BETTER!! Who'd have thought taking volume OFF your chest would make you feel better?? Then, he added 100 cc's to each of my expanders, so I no longer look like I'm 12 years old!! Bonus!

Then we were off to Dr. B's office. He said that everything looked great and gave me a script for some more good drugs. Hopefully after I get through all of this, you won't be seeing me on Celebrity Rehab with Gary Busey (doesn't he look AWFUL??). I see how it can happen. I haven't been taking them during the day because I don't want to be on the phone training a finance manager at a car dealership drooling all over myself. Besides that, if you are off your game talking to some of these guys, THEY WILL EAT YOU ALIVE. So I save the "good stuff" for bedtime. I should be able to sleep really well tonight with a whole lot less pain, which is a total plus.

I want to thank my great friend Jill for coming over Saturday and cleaning my house! What a huge help. Now that I have some better range of motion, I can clean my own toilets, Jill! Either that, or I can bribe the kids with more allowance or a visit to Chuck E. Cheese to do the toilets. Mmm. I think when you bring your kids to Chuck E. Cheese, they should have an Excedrin dispenser for parents right next to the coin dispenser for games! Talk about sensory overload.

Thank you so much Diane D. for agreeing to take Abe for the duration. Diane had a "dry run" with Abe on Sunday and it went well with her family, her dog, and Abe. So Diane is going to take Abe starting this weekend. She lives close by, so we can go visit him so he doesn't think we have abandoned him. I know he will be happy to have another dog to play with because his current ALL DAY hobby is sleeping. I have to say that it is pretty amazing that a dog can sleep for 22 hours a day and still have enough energy to eat a loaf of bread off your counter in two gulps and still leave the paper the bread came in!

I am going to make an appointment for next week to get fitted for a wig. I have to check and see if my insurance company will cover a "cranial prosthesis." Who thinks this stuff up anyway? What it really comes down to is a scratchy rat on your head. I just need to figure out which rat I like the best!

I hope this note finds you all happy, healthy and warm. Three weeks from tomorrow I start my chemo, so I am doing my best to stay healthy and strong before I have all the toxins floating in my bod. I'm sure I will be just fine through my treatments. I am a little freaked about being bald, with no eyebrows and no eyelashes. At least I won't have to worry about poking myself in the eye with my mascara wand for a while!

Love to all, Connie

Abe was back after his two week hiatus. He was sent packing after marking his territory all over the house of the woman who was helping us out. A couple of my friends offered to give Abe a whirl at their houses, and much to my chagrin, he was back because he was a urinating machine. He returned home after his adventures, sans any peeing incidents. Animals are so tuned in to what is going on. I think he knew I was sick because he clung close to me like a one hundred pound hemorrhoid.

God, I'm tired. And I haven't even started chemotherapy yet. My breast surgeon told me after my mastectomies that I was 95 percent done with my treatment. Well, I want to march straight to his office and tell him that he is totally full of shit. Where is he when I lie awake every night contemplating my imminent future? As a matter of fact, where is anyone (namely Mark) while I lie away thinking, thinking, THINKING every night? The constant worry of my relationship with him is almost as exhausting as the cancer.

Chapter 12

Laughter and Toilet Brushes

Friday, January 23, 2009 5:33 PM, CST

I HAVE AMAZING FRIENDS! I am so incredibly blessed! My friends Joan and Brit drove 2 1/2 hrs up from Connecticut today. We were all Mary Kay Directors and always had so much fun when we went to MK events! They brought me lunch, pre-made meals for me and the kids, cleaned my house and made me laugh so hard I almost peed my pants!! What fun we had today!! Thank you so much Joan and Britt!! Joan, I will send you the "toilet brush" next time I go shopping. LOL!!!

I'm feeling pretty good today. I just have been sooo tired. But I'm still spunky! I remember in the first trimester of pregnancy wanting to go to bed every night at 7. Lately, I have been feeling like that ALL DAY LONG. This too shall pass. I keep thinking ahead to June, when I will be done with all of my treatments and regain much needed energy!

The feeling is starting to come back in my arm. It is painful, but at least I am getting feeling back (Thank God for good narcotics!). I am still working on range of motion in my left arm, which seems to be getting better. I have no feeling in my armpit area which makes putting deodorant on a comical challenge. Is it on?? It's very strange.

My friend Amy decided when I was first diagnosed that we needed to have a girls' trip when I recovered, naming the trip "How Connie Got Her Boobs Back." Like, How *Stella Got Her Groove Back*. So today, Joan, Brit and I decided that we are going to Phoenix with some friends for the boob trip. Something to really look forward to.

I met with two wonderful women today, Sue and Suzanne (the Sue Crew), who have the same oncologist as me. We met for coffee and they told me all of the ins and outs of chemo. What to expect, how long it takes, how I will feel, etc. It is remarkable to me how women who go through this challenge (and it IS a challenge) reach out to others and help them through the same struggle. Thanks Sue and Suzanne! Even though this is a tough time in my life, I know that this is a growth experience and I will come out stronger on the other side. The Sue Crew definitely proved that to be true.

Thanks again for all of your phone calls, messages, cards and well wishes! I appreciate all of you.

Life is short, so be HAPPY!!

Love, Connie

I have to say, "Thank god for all of my friends!" I love to laugh: it is by far the best medicine for any situation, especially the predicament I find myself in as of late.

Two of my friends from Connecticut came up to visit me, brought me some dinners that I could easily assemble and offered to clean my house. I am very particular about my house. I like things squeaky clean, to the point of being what I might call anal. Even with a chocolate lab who sheds more than five alpacas, my house is clean. In my ill state, I haven't really been on top of it. I am grateful to my friends for the offer, and they get right to it. They fill my glass with red wine, prop up my feet and commence with cleaning.

It's late in the day and I am still technically working. My phone rings and I answer, handling a work situation while my friend Joan yells from upstairs, "Hey Con! I'm really digging this toilet brush!" Again, Alan Funt is somewhere, because the guy on the other end of the phone says, "Huh? Is someone talking about a toilet?" Needless to say, that fabulous toilet brush turns out to be something I clean the bathroom floor with, not meant for use in a toilet. Oh, it's funny how the silliest of things can make you laugh!

I have had the privilege to meet extraordinary people in my life. Having cancer throws you into a club of sorts. People who are survivors, and others who are fighting the daily grind of cancer to survive. I was truly blessed during my journey to have met two amazing women, who I fondly call "The Sue Crew." Without them, my cancer travels would have taken me on much darker roads. It is important to have connections with people who have already taken the journey. A guided beacon of light is invaluable to tell you what to expect, where the forks are in the road. Everyone's journey is different; a stop sign for some is a yield for others. We all hope to arrive at the same destination—that of wellness.

Chapter 13
Pissy Pants

Monday, January 26, 2009 7:47 PM, CST

I know that "God only gives you what you can handle," but seriously, am I on *Candid Camera*??? I went to see my oncologist today where I found out that my CAT scan and bone scan were free of metastatic breast cancer, BUT, I have a nodule on my thyroid that needs to be looked into. It is unrelated to my breast cancer (thank goodness), but still needs to be further investigated. So another biopsy and possible removal. I must have been a mean cat in a past life or something. My Mom always used to say, "Things always have a way of working themselves out." I know this to be true, but I am reaching the end of my proverbial rope.

After Mark and I met with my oncologist, we met with the chemo nurse for my "chemo education." They need to rename it, "Too Much Information So Your Head Will Explode Toxic Education." This drug will make you feel nauseous, cause you to lose your hair, lower your white and red blood cell count, cause fatigue, weight gain/weight loss, decrease heart function, make your urine RED (as opposed to the previous GREEN), possibly give you mouth sores, blah, blah, blah. Sounds like a BLAST! SIGN ME UP!

OK, so I'm a little pissy today. I'll get over it. And what kills me is that they give you a whole bunch of drugs BEFORE you get the really bad drugs to offset the "badness." I left with a bunch of scripts for nausea and had to laugh at the worst case "suppository" anti-nausea medication (in case the nausea gets too bad). Well I can assure you that the nausea will never get THAT BAD that I will need to use a suppository anti-nausea medication! Are they SERIOUS??

Then I went to my surgeon's office and met with the PA. We talked about my arm pain. Hopefully it will get better, but I may have to have an ultrasound to check on a vein in my arm. But to be honest, I totally wasn't listening because my head was at the oncologist's office rerunning the "toxic chemical education/horrible nausea suppository" scenario. He is going to check with Dr. B about the arm pain and call me tomorrow morning. I should be on my game enough tomorrow to absorb the information when he calls back :)

I was able to set up my schedule for the first 2 cycles (2 treatments with the off week for bloodwork). Mark thought it might be funny to order me a male stripper for my first chemo, but then we got laughing about all of the older men and women in the chemotherapy room stroking out from the shock. Well, the idea was fun.

I made an appointment to get fitted for a wig on Friday afternoon which should be a total adventure. I am going to make a day of it with some girlfriends and get drinks IMMEDIATELY afterward and dinner to celebrate my new "look." On the bright side, I can be someone totally different. Well, let's be honest, I will be someone totally different—I won't have any eyebrows or eye lashes.

Tomorrow I will see my plastic surgeon to get my chest "pumped up." It's like being Stretch Armstrong, but in a different region! Last time I was there, he told me, "you won't be a Dolly Parton and you won't be a Twiggy." Well that certainly leaves a range! And then his nurse followed it up by saying, "Yeah, and you won't have their money either!" LOL! So much for my dollar and a dream!

I keep telling myself, "I will be fine. I will feel better soon. I am in a great mood. OK, I'm a little pissy today. I will beat this thing. I AM NOT TIRED. I will laugh and have fun NO MATTER WHAT. I will get through this. The kids will get through this and be OK." So lots of stuff I am "telling" myself. Maybe I am Sybil.

Well, I hope you all are well. Thanks for all of the phone calls, cards, messages, emails, you know—all of it!! Much love, Connie :)

Thursday, January 29, 2009 3:53 PM, CST

Hey, Sybil!! I'm thinking about you and still here if you need me. I am really hoping the thyroid thing is a benign cyst. They are relatively common. Today is Thursday, so you must know the answer to that by now.

I used Zofran for the nausea and a mouth gel called Hurricane Gel for mouth sores. Both were very good.

So, are you going blonde or red for your new hair look? The wigs are hot sometimes, but your head may get cold from no hair, so it balances out! HA!

Love you much, Mrs. G.

Thursday, January 29, 2009 4:03 PM, CST

You're not Sybil...LOL...that movie is so sick and twisted!! Well, I think this thing with your thyroid is going to turn out fine. I know a girl who had something growing on hers and it was just a lump that had no purpose, so they just took it out. I know you really DO NOT need to go through more surgery right now, but you probably won't have to. As for your wig, I think you should get a blonde one, you've always looked fabulous as a blonde. And blondes have more fun! Trust me, I am one...LOL Love, Kate D.

Thursday, January 29, 2009 8:13 PM, CST

Connie—I know you are going through sooo much right now!!! —Continue to hold on to your friends and family—they want to help in anyway they can!!!!! —Glad you found a great place for your dog!! I'm sure that was a tough decision...Keep up your positive outlook...it will help!!!!!!!!!!!!!! You can have a bad day—everyone does!! —It's OK to not be happy-happy-happy 24/7...I continue to keep you in my prayers!!!! Lots of Love, Liz

Saturday, January 31, 2009 10:25 AM, CST

Connie,

I know we haven't talked in awhile and lately you have been on my mind. I thank God that for some reason I found the sisters on Facebook and Sue Ann told me about the group. I have been searching for your number and I couldn't find it but here you are! Your strength and support from your loving family and friends will get you through this. I want you to know you are in my prayers and I love you!

Karielynn S.

*My dear friend Karielynn from college. My funny sweet sorority sister, who just a year after this entry, died in her sleep. Much love to you Cricket, wherever you may be.

My head is reeling. Stage II-A breast cancer, estrogen-receptor positive, Adriamycin, Cytoxan, Taxol, Tamoxifen, Neulasta shots, anti-nausea medicines, side effects, on and on and freaking on. Holy shit! How much can a person process in an hour?

As a kid, you sit in History class listening to your teacher go on for an hour or more about some figure in history. At the time, you couldn't give a rat's ass because it wasn't happening to YOU! As I sit at the oncologist's office that day listening to the nurse go on for an hour about chemo, I think, "This is going to be MY history!" It is a path I HAVE to take. If I don't, I will BE history. What really throws me for a loop is that there is a *Breast Cancer Dictionary*, courtesy of the American Cancer Society. I read it cover to cover, memorizing the definitions and descriptions as if I were studying for a vocabulary test. Knowledge is power! Or is it a pathway to self-destruction?

According to the American Cancer Society, invasive ductal carcinoma is "a cancer that starts in the milk passages (ducts) of the breast and then breaks through the duct wall, where it invades the fatty tissue of the breast: when it reaches this point, it has the potential to spread (metastasize) elsewhere in the breast, as well as to other parts of the body through the bloodstream and lymphatic system. Invasive ductal carcinoma is the most common type of breast cancer, accounting for about 80% of breast malignancies." Well, at least I have the "popular" kind! I read this over and over, all the while imagining some small cell traveling from my breast to places unknown in my body, like the *Mr. Slim Goodbody* Show we watched on TV as kids, where Mr. Goodbody wore his body suit made to show us how our insides worked.

I have never been one who actively pursues a pity party for myself, but I'm pretty damn close. How does one ever prepare for this illness? It's not like there's a "How To Gear Up For A Breast Cancer Diagnosis" handbook that you can turn to page sixteen for the answer. When you are diagnosed, there are many resources available to answer your questions. But the cancer jargon is overwhelming and more than a bit daunting. There are many support groups you can join, and if that's your thing, more power to you. I decided early on that I didn't want to sit around talking about it all the time. Weekly reports with those less fortunate in prognosis would be the death of me. I had to look forward at my own journey and put my blinders on to others. This may sound completely selfish, but I had to think of my own mental survival, and more importantly, the mental survival of my young children. I decided early on that I would be "up" if it killed me. "Fake it till you make it."

So when I heard the news of my thyroid situation, I thought, "What next? How many more pokes and prods do I have ahead?" There is a point along this cancer journey where you succumb to it. Not in an "I'm going to die" sort of way, but in a way that allows you to move forward, rolling with the punches instead of looking for someone to fight. Don't get me wrong, I was fighting, but I wasn't expending any more energy than necessary to do battle.

And seriously, how many times can I go to the doctor? Don't most people go once or twice a year? WTF, I'm going like EVERY DAY! This is all getting old, and unfortunately, so am I. I feel like this cancer sentence has aged me ten years in the last few weeks.

I'm back to the thought of baldness. It is unbelievable how that has become my focus, and not in a good way. Early on, when I was told the whole story of my mastectomies, I was OBSESSED with the thought of losing my nipples. I couldn't stop thinking about it. How weird was I going to look without nipples? Would my chest have any sensation? Blah, blah, blah. Now, my new obsession is my hair and lack thereof. How am I going to look? Will people think I am a freak? Will anyone really KNOW if I wear my wig? My mind is exhausted and so am I.

I think back to when I was married. How many times I went to bed angry because my ex would do something, or not do something that would send me into a mental frenzy. I would lie there so mad , but what was I really solving? I was married to someone who was impervious to reason, so why say anything? These same thoughts crossed my mind when it came to my cancer. Who was I pissed at? Who would listen, and more important, who would give a shit? Surely, all of my friends and family cared, but who was going to solve the problem?

Therein lies the battle. Who am I fighting with? My cancer? My oncologist? Myself? When I got the news of my possible thyroid cancer, it was then that I realized there was no sense in fighting an internal battle any longer. It was energy I could expend on other things. The mind is a terrible thing to waste, but it is also an "enemy of the state" for those who choose to allow thoughts to fester.

I remember as a kid the "Say No To Drugs" campaign. A guy in a commercial takes an egg and says, "This is your brain," and then breaks the egg over a hot skillet and says, "This is your brain on drugs." I wish I could pluck the cancer from me and throw it into the skillet and watch it burn, along with all of my thoughts.

Chapter 14
The One-Titted Wonder

Sunday, February 1, 2009 8:46 AM, CST

If there is one life lesson to be learned from all of this, it is that you need to live for each day. Which, for me, the "perpetual planner," is a bit difficult. When am I going to be done with this? When am I going to be healthy again? Blah, blah. I do appreciate each day, I just like to know how things are going to turn out. Me and a crystal ball would be BFF's!!

Last Wednesday I got the news that I will most likely need a biopsy of the nodule on my thyroid. I am just waiting for confirmation from my oncologist. Not a HUGE deal, but it's just ONE MORE THING to deal with. When my oncologist told me about this last week, I asked him to leave the room, come back and tell me something better (or preferably just start over and not tell me anything bad). I also told him that he is on my "s list" and the s doesn't stand for SPECIAL like he thinks!

On Thursday I noticed that my right breast was red and hot and painful, even though I really don't have any feeling there (weird). I didn't want to complain about it, so I ice packed it to see what happens. By Thursday night, I had a fever and feel like crap, so I call my plastic surgeon. When the answering service connected us, I said, "It's your favorite patient!" He laughed and told me I needed to start on anti-biotics ASAP and come in and see him the next day.

I tried to get out of going the next day because I was totally slammed with work. The last couple of days in the car busi-ness is a mad dash to the finish. I HAD STUFF TO DO. So I was basically told to GET THERE by the nurse. Friday was wig day, and I had so much to do, so I'm thinking "crap." I get there and he does not look so happy. He draws fluid off my right side, sends it off for culture and informs me that I will most likely need to have the expander removed on Monday to clean out the infection. WHICH MEANS, it's ANOTHER surgery, delayed chemo, having ONE BOOB for months, another surgery to put it back in, more months to expand that side, and a few months delay in getting my new rack. So my little calendar of "when will I be done with this" just keeps getting LONGER.

He sends me over to get pre-op bloodwork and I tell him that I have a very important appointment that afternoon and time is of the essence. He looks at me like, "what could be more important than pre-op bloodwork?" I tell him, "I am getting fitted for a wig, so I have an important appointment with a bunch of dead squirrels." He thinks I'm nuts—no pun intended.

My right side was really bad again yesterday, so I called. He told me to get someone to drive me (so I could take drugs) and drag myself up to his office ASAP. So yesterday, my dear friend Jill took me up and he drained it again. I won't know until I get there tomorrow if I need to have it removed. He has an OR booked at his surgical office with an anesthesiologist just in case. The "planner" in me is beside myself. I will keep you posted.

So the "squirrel fest" on Friday was pretty funny. If my friends Chris, Christine and Rene weren't there, I probably would have cried instead of laughed. Trying on wigs for fun is one thing, but when you know that you will be bald, it takes on a whole new meaning. You have to imagine what you are going to look like every time you leave your house. I have visions of picking my kids up at the indoor soccerplex, walking across a windy parking lot, my hair flying off and chasing after some car that got my "hair" stuck under their wheel. Better not hit a muffler, it will MELT. I had to laugh because the wig lady told me that you have to be careful when you open your oven because the heat from the oven will singe your "hair." Well, there's another visual. Having a bunch of friends over, cooking and just before I open my oven saying, "Wait a minute, I have to take off my wig," get the food out and put my wig back on. What a riot!

I tried on a bunch of wigs. Short ones. Long ones. Elvira ones. We had some laughs. Some wigs are really wiggy looking—like having a SQUIRREL on your head! And then there are others that have an actual "part" that looks like it is coming from your scalp. It actually doesn't look so bad. A little more "poofy" than I would wear, but still not so bad. EXPENSIVE, but not so bad. Having cancer is physically, mentally and emotionally taxing, but it is also costly. Almost like getting a divorce all over again. BONUS!

After the wig hunt, 7 of my good friends and I went out for dinner and drinks. We laughed and laughed, and ate and ate. It was a lot of fun and I really needed to laugh after the latest boob incident. Just like Freud (I think) said, everything "revolves around the boob." The guy knew his stuff.

So tomorrow, I will know more about the infected boob situation. I am on mega doses of two different antibiotics. I am so hoping that this heals itself before tomorrow. Anything can happen, right? At some point, I will catch a break. I hope it is tomorrow.

No matter what happens, I will deal with it and keep smiling and laughing. I have no choice. I hope this note finds you all well. Thanks so much for your well wishes! Keep the good vibes coming. I should be turning a corner here soon!

Love, Connie :)

Sunday, February 1, 2009 8:56 AM, CST

Connie,

It sounds like you still have a wonderful sense of humor, keep it that way. I am sure whatever cards are dealt tomorrow you will do just fine with them. I will pray that it all goes well for you. Keep smiling and think only positive thoughts. Maybe one night this week I will swing by to pay you a visit. Keep your chin up! :)

Sandy D.

Sunday, February 1, 2009 10:29 AM, CST.

Connie, I don't even know what to write at this time. Just hang in there. I am praying that the antibiotics work. I know this all seems like so much and actually it is, but take each step, each day a little at a time. You will make it through. I wish I was there to help you with whatever you need, but since I cannot I will think of you and keep you in my prayers. Keep the laughter, it is your strength that God has given you to get through whatever the next couple of months throws your way. Here's hoping for Great Doses of antibiotic news for tomorrow. Love Judy G.

Sunday, February 1, 2009 1:01 PM, CST

Hey Con,

Hope you got my voicemail today (no worries about calling me back). Sorry again for missing both Friday and Saturday. I did not know you had encountered all these new obstacles, I am sorry to hear about this but I do appreciate you writing about it on here so we all know what is going on. You are my in my prayers.

Take Care and Much Love, Missy T. (and Jamie too!)

Sunday, February 1, 2009 1:07 PM, CST

Connie, you are in my thoughts and prayers. Just know that it is way OK to have "pissy" days. You are more than entitled to them. We all have them, some more than others. I believe that God doesn't give us more than we can handle. He is always with us and in those times when it gets really tough, know that he is with you and will carry you through it. You are so incredibly strong…stronger than you know. I wish that I could be that strong about things in my life. God Bless…Pam R.

Sunday, February 1, 2009 3:38 PM, CST

Hey Connie,

I just read the last update. Are you sure that you were not an English major in school? Your flair with words is truly amazing. I read your entries and laugh and cry all at the same time. I just wanted you to know that I am thinking of you every day. Feel good!

Love,

SueAnn L.

Monday, February 2, 2009 10:36 AM, CST

Connie, you crack me up...I really think you need to save every one of your emails to us and write a short book...I wish I could come up with a snappy name for it...I'll think about it. My stepdad, who seems to have a direct connection with the man upstairs, has been praying for you, and let me tell you when you have my stepdad praying only good things happen...All of these setbacks are just that, if someone tells you that you can't control everything and that you have to learn to go with it...I am so glad that you have wonderful friends that can make you laugh and take good care of you mentally...comedic relief is so important. There are a few books out the by Doctor Bernie Seigel...I think that's how it's spelled. He was an oncologist at Yale New Haven in Connecticut and wrote about how you have to look at Cancer with the humor side...Get the book...If you want, email me and let me know your address if you are interested: I will get it for you...But only if you want it, it's an amazing book that I read while my mom was going through her cancer...I think of you often and pray for you... Take care of you and stay happy and keep on finding the humor in all of this...I love the dead squirrel thing...I am sure you look wonderful...Love ya girl...Laura D.

Monday, February 2, 2009 9:01 PM, CST

Connie,

I'm so sorry to hear about your setback and how deformed you feel. That sucks! Just know I love you even though you're a "one-titted wonder" right now and a wonder you are. I am praying for strength and healing. Man, are you gonna be one strong cookie when you're done with all of this. You're an inspiration to many!

Deana

Monday, February 2, 2009 9:09 PM, CST

Connie, I'm so sorry this rollercoaster you're on keeps throwing dips and whirls at you. I'm praying for you—I love you!

Julie C.

Chapter 15
Squirrel fest

You really find out who your friends are when you face a crisis. The breast cancer is a "stop you in your tracks" crisis, but the wig-finding mission doesn't lag very far behind it. My friends are my "sanity savers" for the wig mission. We arrive at the wig place and I think, "I should have had a cosmopolitan to gear me up for this!" I watch as the woman at the wig place puts different wigs on my head and styles them. It is an out-of-body experience. Surreal. Who is this person looking back at me in the mirror? It certainly isn't ME. I've never felt so far away from myself as I do that afternoon.

I tried on numerous wigs. So many different styles, but I stuck to blonde so I would present the illusion that I was well and just suffering a crisis in style. I was amazed at the number of styles that looked like old lady hair. It brought me back to trips to my mother's hairdresser as a kid.

Every month, usually on a Saturday, we would take the hour long trip to get my mother's hair done. As a kid, the place seemed huge. It was this long narrow salon with barber chairs lining both sides and all male hairdressers. My mom's hairdresser was this white-haired guy named John. I thought it was so cool that he would let me sit in the chair next to his to watch him cut my mother's hair while my brother ran up and down the rows of chairs scaring the shit out of all of the old ladies who came in for a wash and set. Some of the wigs I was looking at looked just like those ladies' hair when they came in for their weekly styling.

My friends all have positive things to say about the wig I choose. After all, it is most like myself. It was a little longer than my old bob, but it fit my face and wasn't quite so "wiggy" as some of the others. I try it on one last time to make sure it is "the one." Unfortunately, that feeling of "This is it!" doesn't wash over me in the same way as finding my wedding dress. I can't believe I am thirty-nine years old and getting a wig to cover what will soon be my bald head. My eyes well up and I am about to lose it. My friend Chris looks at me and says, "Breathe Con. Breathe." I'm breathing! Otherwise I'd be dead, right? Breathing is not helping the overwhelming sense of panic that is rising in my throat.

How did I even find myself here? Is this payback for being a little shit as a kid? Fighting with my brother? Partying in college? OK, I may have overdone it a bit on that one. I can't believe I even got a degree. Is it because that jelly fish stung my boob in St. Maarten and Mark peed on it? Is it a coincidence that my cancer was found in the same breast?

When I was in college, it is probably shocking to know that I earned my beer money with my entrepreneurial zest for cutting guys' hair and chalking licenses. Five bucks a pop. I was rich! I mean, a beer blast was only three dollars! I was rolling in Abe Lincolns! All I had to do was change the 68's and 69's to 65's so we could appear at least 21 instead of 17 and 18. I even had this nifty little white chalking pencil. These days, I'd be arrested and handcuffed to a chair, parched, never making it to the beer blast.

Cutting frat boy hair was my real money maker. Guys can be pretty desperate and, let's face it, they couldn't give a shit if their sides are even. First off, I have NO IDEA how I ever started cutting anyone's hair. Who the hell did I think I was, Paul Mitchell? Anyways, this one frat guy asked me to cut his hair. "Little Tony" they called him. He was Italian (of course) and had kinky black hair. One afternoon, he came knocking on my dorm room door. Thirty minutes later, he was out the door, I'd swept his hair into the hallway, and I was off to take a shower, my little tote of toiletries in hand. I came out of the shower wrapped in a towel and headed for my room. One of the girls on my floor walked towards me with her boyfriend, and as I almost got to my room, her boyfriend's

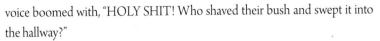

voice boomed with, "HOLY SHIT! Who shaved their bush and swept it into the hallway?"

OH … MY … GOD. I couldn't walk into my room! He'd think I shaved my bush! Maybe I could say it was my roommate. What could I do? I was in a freaking towel! I walked past my room to my friend Larry's room further down the hall. I knocked on his door and as he opened it he said, "This looks interesting." Much to his chagrin, I stayed in my towel until the coast was clear.

If only I could just have a haircut. Instead, I'll soon be sweeping ALL of my hair out into the hallway.

Monday, February 2, 2009 8:25 PM, CST

If "a setback is a setup for a comeback," then LOOK OUT PEOPLE! I had to have the surgery today and have the expander taken out because I had a staph infection in that area. My surgeon thinks that it may be from the expansion he did last Monday, maybe from the needle. Mark is away right now and when I told him what it was, his first reaction was, "What, did they rub your boob all over a gym floor before they stuck the needle in there??" Seriously, how does this happen? No sense trying to figure it out. It happened. Now everything else I have to go through to be done with all of this is just going to take that much longer. This just set me back about 3 months. I have to call my oncologist tomorrow and see about the thyroid situation and see when I can start my chemo. It definitely won't be next week.

I think the hardest thing I am facing right now is that I feel totally deformed. I was feeling pretty good before this because I was having each of the expanders filled gradually and was almost back to my old self. Now I am completely flat on one side. I'm the "one-titted wonder!" I don't even want to look in the mirror.

I will get through this. I'm just not feeling so great about things right now. I'm tired and sore and I've pretty much had it. I'm going to take a pain pill and go to bed. I will keep you all posted.

Love you all, Connie :)

Tuesday, February 3, 2009 7:37 AM, CST

Connie,

I love how you continue to keep your sense of humor through this whole thing. That is what is going to get you through all of this! (and the pain pills, of course). Continue to keep your chin up and lean on your friends for help. My thoughts and prayers are with you.

Elena T.

Tuesday, February 3, 2009 11:36 AM, CST

Hey Connie, So sorry to hear about your setbacks. You seem to have a good attitude and believe me, that's half the battle! Keep in mind that some days are just better than others. And on those rough days (or weeks) try to smile, pop a pain pill, and try to nap. You're in my thoughts and prayers.

Tracey L.

Tuesday, February 3, 2009 3:21 PM, CST

Connie...now I'm pissed that you should have to deal with more of this stuff. There is that saying, "if things can go wrong, they will." I can't believe that the damned needle could cause a staph infection...I thought they were always new...You are blessed to have a great sense of humor but it is sometimes harder to muster up. Keep the "good drugs" on hand for the bad times, and remember, take a nap… nothing is as important as you are and that you are rested. It helps clear the head also. I keep the prayers coming your way and again, whatever I can do for you, please let me know…Stay strong little lady…better days are coming…

Love n prayers…Dotte C.

Mark is away visiting his pregnant sister and her husband. She is having problems with her pregnancy, or so I was told. I remember conversations with Mark that sounded as if he were in a wind tunnel. I would question him about it and he would say he was calling me from the one place on her lawn where his cell phone worked. I'd say, "You have Verizon, doesn't your phone even work in the Holland Tunnel?" Honestly, the stories were ridiculous and he made me feel terrible for wanting him to be home with me while I went through my ordeal. He'd say, "If your brother were going through a health issue, wouldn't you want to be there with him?" So there I was, sick and going through some serious shit, made to feel guilty about wanting who I THOUGHT was my life partner to be with me. I was sick, not stupid.

Many months later, I would stumble onto the lie. The intricacy of the lies. The details were truly astonishing. He had been back in the tropics. With whom, I'll never know. I was betrayed by deceit, denial, and deliberation. Another woman would have been easier to deal with. I'll never know the truth. But I will say this. It was a lonely time in my life. The cancer, the relationship (or lack thereof). There was a palpable void in me that I could not fill. There was only an intermittency of companionship that would later prove to have been a farce.

Then the realization hits of who I am physically. OMG I have one breast. Truly, the one-titted wonder I have now become. Why is it as women we allow ourselves to be defined by our breast size? We wait—similar to watching water boil—for our breasts to finally develop. Little buds that eventually require a training bra. When we emerge onto the bra scene, we've made it (some more than others).

I don't even remember my breasts anymore. Thirty-nine years of the same chest ... erased. I don't even remember what my nipples looked like. Maybe I'll head down to the nearest tattoo parlor and have hot pink gerbera daisies tattooed on my chest when this adventure is over. How will I explain THAT to the next man in my life?

"Um, I wanted to become one with nature so I had my favorite flower tattooed closest to my heart."

"So what happened to your nipples?" he'll ask.

"Well, they were sacrificial lambs on my quest."

Thursday, February 5, 2009 1:17 PM, CST

This has been a tough week, probably the toughest I have had since receiving my diagnosis. I saw my plastic surgeon this morning in hopes of getting my latest drain taken out. NO CAN DO. Fabulous. As it turns out, my staph infection is resistant to the antibiotic I have been on for the last week, so he switched me to a new one today to see how I do.

I must be the WORST patient EVER because I get easily frustrated and do whatever I want instead of listening (surprise!). After my surgery Monday, I was supposed to have stayed wrapped in this uncomfortable, itchy bandage thing until today. Yeah, like that's going to happen. I took it off Monday night. So I show up today wearing a non-bra top (I am tired of being a slave to the surgical bra which looks like an "over the shoulder boulder holder" for women who can't keep themselves upright) and my surgeon looked at me like, "what happened here?" So I told him that it got on my nerves and I took it off and he could take out my drain today or I would go home and do it myself because I am tired of being tired from pain killers and the drain was causing pain and therefore my tiredness. He looked at his nurse like "Oh boy."

My patience is running thin. I was just starting to feel normal before this happened. Like I could get through A DAY and not think about having cancer. I had a chest and thought, "people won't know that I have breast cancer when they look at me." Like, the bald head and no eyebrows won't be a dead giveaway in a couple of weeks! What was I thinking??

My surgeon is sympathetic to my plight. He really is fantastic and thank God he has a great sense of humor. If he was a totally serious guy, he would probably want me in a straightjacket. He negotiated with me to keep the drain in for one more day. So I will get it taken out tomorrow. AND I promised I would stay in the stupid bandage thing until tomorrow. The sacrifices I am making for good health and boobs! Ridiculous!

Next Wednesday I still have my appointment for chemo. I will see my oncologist first and then he will decide if I am going to receive my treatment that day or not. Everything is hinging on how well I do on this antibiotic and if the staph infection disappears. The situation I am in is rare (figures) and I didn't realize quite how serious this kind of infection can be. My plastic surgeon told me today that I am definitely earning my boobs with all of the hoopla I am going through. No kidding. They better be SPECTACULAR when this is all over or we are going to have words!

I hope everyone is doing well. Thank you all so much for the lovely cards, emails, messages and phone calls. I am trying to keep my meltdowns to a minimum, realizing that laughter really is the best medicine!

Keep smiling! Love, Connie :)

Thursday, February 5, 2009 1:01 PM, CST

Hey Connie, You know what always helps? A big, huge, hot fudge sundae…

Kate D.

Thursday, February 5, 2009 1:37 PM, CST

OK, listen here…The doc says keep things on or in for a reason, I know from past surgeries, that things are told and done for a reason…I know this sounds harsh and yes, easier said than done. But for God sakes they have protocols for these things…Please, I beg of you to listen to them…Now as for you on the edge of meltdowns, perhaps writing these emails more often is a good release for you…Then again, maybe not. But know that you are not in this alone and there are a lot of people who love you and care for you, and all of this will be behind you sooner than you think…Enjoy the days you look like and feel like crap cause that gives you a reason to act crappy and be crappy…And no one will bust your ass about it…But just think, around the corner is health and beauty and a wonderful outlook on life as you know it…I love ya and think about you. Praying for you…Laura D.

Thursday, February 5, 2009 2:18 PM, CST

Connie,

Just wanted to let you know that I am thinking of you. (((hugs)))

SueAnn L.

Thursday, February 5, 2009 3:17 PM, CST

Connie,

Thinking of you…

xo Missy T.

Thursday, February 5, 2009 4:08 PM, CST

Hi Connie,

I think of you every evening and send loving, healing thoughts your way. So sorry you have a staph infection. You will get through this—it's one day at a time. Love You, Maureen L.

Thursday, February 5, 2009 5:41 PM, CST

Connie, I am so sorry you got one of the resistant kinds of infections. Please keep the drain in as long as the doctor feels is needed. Let it drain out all the bad stuff in there. Better out than in. All of these setbacks are a real PIA I'm sure, but your sense of humor will get you through. I think about you every day and look forward to these updates. Take each day one at a time and celebrate that you got through one more today and then tomorrow, etc. It means one more day closer to recovery. You are in my prayers. Love Judy G.

Thursday, February 5, 2009 5:43 PM, CST

Miss Connie, God love ya!! So sorry to hear about all your setbacks. As difficult as it is for you, you have a lot of friends and people who love you and are rooting for you!! I still keep you in my thoughts and prayers. Just take things one day at a time and hang in there. You will get through this!!!

Keep up your positive attitude and great sense of humor. All the best... Debbie D.

Chapter 16
Scars and A Little Self-Loathing

I caught a glimpse of myself in the mirror as I got out of the shower one day. Nude flesh from the neck down, scars diagonal across my chest on both sides. My very own scarlet letter, a hieroglyphics version that I pray will fade. I think then of my mother's scar from her own mastectomy. How had she felt? No reconstruction, just an L-shaped scar, a constant reminder of her own mortality.

I look at my scars and am reminded of much the same, but know that eventually, I will be restored on some level. I will never be what I was before the cancer, but somehow, I think, I will be better. Better in the sense that I have looked death in the face and kicked its ass. I know that I have a long journey ahead and I am mentally preparing myself for the ride.

Sometimes I think it would be great if I could just sleep until the journey is over. Then I won't feel a thing. I can be a spectator in my own life for a bit. Much like my ex-husband during our marriage. But the reality is that if I don't actually FACE IT, then what am I really going to gain from the journey? Months from now, I wouldn't be able to look someone in the eye who is about to embark on the same painful adventure and be relatable. There has to be a reason I am dealing with this, and not just because of my genetic predisposition.

I look at that damn drain hanging from my chest. I have to hold it up as I get dressed because it hurts like hell when it just hangs there, stitched to my side much the same as the garden hose attached to my house. Said hose will later be run over with my snow blower the following winter.

Friday, February 6, 2009 8:06 PM, CST

The drain is OUT!! I have to say that it is just not natural to have tubes sticking out of your chest. Not to mention, that it is completely uncomfortable!

I told my plastic surgeon today that after everything I have been going through with the boob situation, I better be getting a HUGE discount on liposuction! He said, "ABSOLUTELY!" I'll have to check back on that when I'm done with the boob job :)

You never realize until you are in a health crisis just how much you tend to take your good health for granted. Bitching and complaining over the little things in life just seems so stupid now. Who cares if there are clothes all over or the beds aren't made? It's not like Martha Stewart's coming over. You can't sweat the small stuff. I try this approach to things, but I still fight myself mentally about cleaning up. Then my tiredness wins out and I grab a bowl of ice cream and head for the couch. This, I know, will catch up with me (the eating ice cream bit).

Everyday I think we need to look at where we are and be grateful. I saw the story of a woman on *Oprah* this week who went into the hospital to give birth to her second child, ended up having some infection that caused her limbs to turn black and they had to be amputated. This INCREDIBLE woman is such an inspiration. With prosthetics and pure

WILL she is a wife and mother and cares for her family. Her story was truly amazing.

And just an hour before watching that show I had one of my five-minute meltdowns about not having boobs! I felt like a complete IDIOT! A selfish moron. Amidst all of this crap I am dealing with, I can do the small things. Like paint Alyssa's nails, braid her hair, help Alex put his Legos together. What's worse is that sometimes I DON'T FEEL like doing these things (horrible mother), and I think about this woman who would give ANYTHING to be able to do what I and so many of us can do every day. So basically, I tell myself, BUCK UP AND DEAL!

I am grateful for where I am even if I'm not where I want to be. I would like to be able to extend my left arm all the way, but I can't since my lymph node surgery. It's painful, but I am going to start physical therapy so it will get better (I'm hoping). My chest looks like a cross between a 12 year old girl on one side and a 7 year old boy on the other side. I don't want to look at it, but I know that eventually that will get better too. I will lose my hair, but that will grow back. IT WILL ALL GET BETTER. I know this. But I keep thinking about that woman who doesn't have easy fixes to her physical problems. It just makes you think.

I am one lucky chick to have the love and support of so many people. I want to thank you all for that. I appreciate all of the cards, messages, visits, calls, meals, prayers and positive thoughts. You are all carrying me through this.

Thanks for being there! Love, Connie :)

Friday, February 6, 2009 11:54 AM, CST

Connie,

Just want to let you know I am thinking of you constantly and if anyone can get past this next hurdle it is you! You are one amazing woman and your strength and attitude are so remarkable! I'm planning a trip out your way in March and would love to come and see you and also drop off a bunch of meals for you and the kids. I love you Connie and will talk to you soon.

Love, Lainey H.

Friday, February 6, 2009 9:14 PM, CST

Hey Connie,

You're so right, we do take things for granted...so many things. Thank you for all your positive thinking, and thank you Connie for reminding me how thankful I am for my children, grandchildren, and my health.

Love you

Debra D.

Saturday, February 7, 2009 8:14 AM, CST

Hey Connie,

Like I said yesterday, you are a true inspiration to us all. You are right, you will get through this. You are one amazing lady! It was good to see you yesterday. Once you have your plan in motion, please e-mail me and let me know what areas you need help in that week.

Love ya Claire D.

Saturday, February 7, 2009 9:43 AM, CST

I have to tell you, reading your emails inspired me. To know that you are going through what you are going through and still able to find the humor is a wonderful thing. God Bless you for that. I, on the other hand, would be a total basket case. I find your strength and FORTITUDE amazing. I hope and pray if and when I am faced with whatever life throws my way that I will remember your emails and your humor… Love you girl and keep it up…Please please know that you are being prayed for and you will make it through this like you have made it through other things…Grow from this… Many hugs…Laura D.

Saturday, February 7, 2009 12:33 PM, CST

Hi Connie, You are truly an inspiration to so many of us!!! Writing your journal entries is so healthy for you. You can really express yourself and give all of us a vision of what you are feeling, how we can help and embrace you with love and support. I'm here, you know that always. See you soon. Love, Chris F.

I truly believe that laughter is the best medicine. I laugh a lot and throughout my illness, laughter was a critical component to my sanity. Every weekday at 4pm, I would watch *The Ellen DeGeneres Show*. It was an hour of much-needed escape that I treasured almost daily. A brief timeslot in my day to forget about feeling like crap and to laugh at someone who had the ability to laugh at herself, a kinship I shared.

One afternoon, I turned it on to find a repeat episode. I had already had my laughs so I turned my attention to Oprah. Oprah always speaks of her "aha moments," epiphanies of the heart. My mother always told me that you have to appreciate what you have and know that many others are in worse places in their lives than where you may find yourself in a single moment. I will never forget this particular day. It was MY "aha moment."

The story of this woman on *Oprah* was nothing short of inspiring. Physical adversity was not in her repertoire, only a conviction to live her life with purpose. To be the best mother she could be to her children. A role I shared, but did I take for granted? So what if I had one breast at the moment? I was able to put Legos together with my son and paint my daughter's fingernails. I sat on my bed and cried watching this woman's story. Not in pity, but in disappointment with my own thoughts and feelings. How could I, at any moment along this journey, feel sorry for myself?

The human spirit can never be suppressed: it is meant to soar. My "aha moment" comes from knowing that you have to dig deep within yourself to know your purpose. It was then that I knew I would make it through this mess because my purpose was my children. To teach them how to be loving, giving people who persevere no matter what life throws at them. How many nights did I lie awake thinking, "What if this gets me like it got my mother?" No longer would I allow my head to go there. It was a dark place I didn't want to travel to again. My fear would not win this battle. My will to survive was going to win the war.

To this day, I think of this woman and her strength often. If I were ever to have the honor of meeting her, I think how grateful I would be to tell her that she changed my life that day. I truly believe that you see things when you need to see them.

That day, my vision was crystal clear.

Chapter 17
Orange Pee

Wednesday, February 11, 2009 6:40 PM, CST

One treatment down, seven more to go!! I went in for the chemo today not knowing if I was going to receive it or not because of my recent infection/surgery. My blood counts were good, so I got the go-ahead.

There is such a fine line between the dread of knowing something is going to happen and the acceptance of it actually happening. The only thing I can even come close to comparing it to is your first pregnancy. You are so excited, amazed at the process and then at about eight months you realize, "S%$T, this kid has to come out!" Then you give birth, and say "Oh, I'd do that again" and most of us do. The difference with chemo is that you don't have a bundle of joy in the end but (hopefully) good health.

So the process is interesting to say the least. Having a port in my chest is not fun, but I guess it beats a needle in the arm over and over and over. The only thing is, the chemo nurse sticks the needle STRAIGHT IN, not at any sort of an angle. There was a near "pass out" moment from that for me and my dear friend Lisa who took me today. Now we're prepared. I received a couple of anti-nausea meds in the IV first and then the first part of my chemo which is a red liquid (Adriamycin). Makes your pee orange, another BONUS! It started in my IV and felt like a million ants were running all over my head. It lasted about a minute, but it was a minute too long. Really creepy. After that, I got the second half of my treatment (Cytoxan I think) by IV over the course of half an hour. All in all, it wasn't so bad. The nurse told me I will start to feel crappy in 24 to 36 hours.

Tomorrow I have to go back and have my $7000 shot of Neulasta. Isn't that CRAZY?? What's even more crazy, is that I need 8 of them! $56,000 in shots! I AM high maintenance! So the shot is to boost my red and white blood cell counts and I have been told it will be quite painful to my bones and joints once it gets through my system. That compounded with nausea and fatigue, I ought to be Polly Freakin Anna!

My oncologist told me today to expect to be bald (or close to bald) when I go back for my next treatment in two weeks. I have to order my wig on Friday, and at the first sign of hair loss, I'm buzzing it all off. The kids want to be a part of the buzzing. Maybe Alex wants revenge for all of the buzz cuts I've given him! I'll have some friends come over and with the kids there, I won't be able to have a meltdown. Instead of GI Jane, I can be GI Connie. I will be Kojak's midget twin!

I got the news about my thyroid today. I not only have a cyst on the left side of my thyroid, but I got lucky and they found one to match on the right side! My oncologist said that they will have to be addressed (removed), but he wants me to get through my chemo and then we'll deal with it.

If I think about all of this—the chemo, being bald, the thyroid, the 2+ surgeries left to reconstruct my breasts, a possible hysterectomy—I just want to crawl in a hole with a blanket and a big-ass bowl of ice cream. It is overwhelming. So right now, I just want to think about getting through this week with the chemo, the shot, and hopefully not feeling too much like crap.

Before I forget, I want to thank the person who sent me chocolate-covered strawberries. They are one of my addictions! THANK YOU SO MUCH!!

Thanks again for all of your thoughts and prayers! I am keeping a stiff upper lip. Hopefully, I can keep it stiff enough so I don't hurl! I'll keep you posted!

Love, Connie :)

Wednesday, February 11, 2009 8:28 PM, CST

HI Connie, I just wanted to send you a BIG HUG and let you know that I think of you every day and pray for you to keep your positive attitude, strength and determination going. Rest and take care of yourself. I'll talk to you soon. Call me if you need me. I can cook, clean and even do your windows!!!! Love you, Chris F.

Wednesday, February 11, 2009 8:32 PM, CST

You are the bravest woman I have ever known in my life and although this situation is not funny at all I still find myself laughing every time I read your blog ...I would love to be there for GI CONSTANCE!!!!! Love you and miss you. Let me know when you are feeling up for visitors!!! Talk with you soon Connie

I love you !!! Andrea G.

Wednesday, February 11, 2009 9:01 PM, CST

One down! I'm so glad you didn't have to postpone. That much closer to being done. You are so brave; you really are an inspiration to all of us. My friend at work just went through this, and it was around 2 weeks that she lost her hair. She wears her wig or really cool scarves and looks awesome. You will too. Put me on your schedule to take you to your treatment. Let me know anything you need this week. Take care of yourself! Talk to you soon!

Love,

Mary Beth F.

Wednesday, February 11, 2009 9:23 PM, CST

Connie,

Here's to only 7 more treatments. It means just that much closer to being done. Hang tough. The rough part is ahead and don't be too hard on yourself if you do feel like crap. These meds are made for you to feel that way. I know you got prescriptions for other meds. I hope you filled them and will take them to help get through. I think about you all the time and I pray that you get by one day at a time. Keep the humor going. GI Connie here we go. Please keep us informed, and if you need a pick-me-up please call. I would love to call you, but am afraid I will catch you at a bad time. Love ya my old roomie. Judy G.

Thursday, February 12, 2009 6:56 AM, CST

Hey GI Connie—the next time you go for treatment ask if there is anything that will make you pee purple. You'd be the first AD (Alpha Delta Theta, my sorority) to accomplish that—or at least I think you would be! Who knows with all the crap we used to drink downtown. I think of you and pray for you every day. Hope to see you soon. Love, Margaret C.

Thursday, February 12, 2009 8:01 AM, CST

Con—I only know that God has something very special planned for you to have you go through so much suffering. I know this must be a very scary time and I hope you can feel this big hug I'm giving you right now. I always have known that you are such a special person with a spirit, drive and enthusiasm...courage and strength that far surpasses anyone I have ever known. I love you, pray for you and send lots of positive Karma your way, every day.

Hang in there girlfriend—only 7 more to go...

Luv ya

Kathy S.

Thursday, February 12, 2009 9:54 AM, CST

Connie...another day, another hurdle...it's good that you still have your wonderful sense of humor...you are such a terrific lady. I would love to attend the "buzz cut session" Do you think your daughter will want one too? Maybe we girls should all do it for you...what a trip that would be...the towns would think that the Hari Krishna's were back (can't spell that name very well) You are truly a "piece of work."

I'm praying for you each day and I hope the chemo gets easier. We will talk soon...I will call you.

Dotte C.

Thursday, February 12, 2009 12:41 PM, CST

Hey Connie,

Just a quick note to let you know that I am thinking about you...stay strong...I want to drink a beer with you at Homecoming!!

Lauren J.

Thursday, February 12, 2009 4:07 PM, CST

7 more treatments to go...should we try and make a song about it like pledging?? Thinking of you often Connie. If you need anything, you know where I am! I like what Lauren says...we need to drink some beer in Oct.

Love ya!

SueAnn L.

Thursday, February 12, 2009 4:33 PM, CST

Connie, I think about you every day! I truly admire your courage and sense of humor. I heard you and Joan had a great time together! Please let me know if I can help you out in any way. I'd be more than happy to drive you to any of your appointments or whatever. Keep your spirit. You really are a special person.

Lisa C.

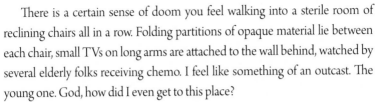

There is a certain sense of doom you feel walking into a sterile room of reclining chairs all in a row. Folding partitions of opaque material lie between each chair, small TVs on long arms are attached to the wall behind, watched by several elderly folks receiving chemo. I feel like something of an outcast. The young one. God, how did I even get to this place?

"Let's get this over with," I think. Lisa sits down in the chair next to me and the nurse approaches in this HAZMAT-looking suit and I'm thinking "What the hell is with this getup?" The nurse informs me that it prevents the chemotherapy from getting onto her skin. The nurses need to avoid skin contact with it and yet it is going straight into MY VEINS?!

The anxiety and anticipation of chemotherapy is hard to put into words. If I can just get through these next three hours, I will have one down and seven more to go. I am forced to think this way because it is the only way I can survive it. It's not like I can spend one whole day receiving all the chemo and get it the hell over with (like I used to hammer out fifteen-page college papers the night before they were due). This required time, the spacing of treatments and patience I would learn to acquire.

Now, I am a planner. I like to know the outcome of things—a very difficult characteristic to break free of while having cancer. A character flaw, if you will. Just knowing what to expect weakens the anxiety. I have a basic idea of what to expect with this chemo. What I DID NOT expect, was the feeling of fire ants in my crotch and in my hair with the first part of the treatment. OMG, this is nuts! Do I say anything? Breathe, Connie, breathe.

The second half of the treatment takes longer. The bag of clear poison hangs on an IV post dripping one drip at a time into my chest. I close my eyes and strain to hear the drops so I can count them. I lose track after thirty. I'm too tired to count and really, who gives a rat's ass HOW MANY drops it takes to empty the bag? It's not like I'm going to look over at the old guy next to me and say, "Hey, I've had more drops than you."

I arrive home after my chemo, get out of the car and think, "Maybe this won't be so bad." Mark was coming over for dinner and staying the night, so if the dreaded expectant puking were to arrive, I would have someone to hold what little hairs I had on my head as I prayed to the porcelain god.

I decide to cheat and make a boxed dinner with added chicken for my first post-chemo meal. Mark helps me and adds 20,000 dashes of pepper. All I can think is, "Stop it with the fucking pepper!" So we sit down to eat and I say, "Would you like some chicken with your pepper?" OMG, I am going to be a total rag-picker on chemo!

I wonder if I am the first chemo patient to want to have sex after having chemo? As Mark and I go at it, I have one of the moments where you (may) run your grocery list through your mind, but instead I think, "I wonder if all of this physical 'activity' will make the chemo run through my veins faster?"

We decide to watch a movie afterwards, some stupid sci-fi flick. I watch some mechanical arachnoid chasing after a kid in torn jeans and think that I am starting to feel as if I have been squished like a bug. I take an anti-nausea pill to ward off all signs of impending illness and go to bed.

Chapter 18
The First Aftermath

Sunday, February 15, 2009 10:46 AM, CST

Well, I seem to have made it through my first treatment. My "stiff upper lip" theory didn't quite make it. Aside from becoming one with the porcelain god yesterday morning, I seem to have come through this unscathed.

I cannot remember ever sleeping so much in my life. Take a pill, sleep. Take a pill, sleep. Almost like drinking till 4 in the morning in college and sleeping till 2 in the afternoon. My mother could never quite understand that logic. Who sleeps past noon??

So today, day 4 after chemo, I am feeling normal, although what is my normal? I have to take a break from being the schizoid cleaner I usually am. What's a few dust bunnies? As long as they don't get up and HOP, who cares?

I am going to order my wig tomorrow. And just so I don't have a freak fest over losing my hair, I may shave my head once I get it. I know I will be bald by my next treatment, so I have been checking my pillow case every morning like a lunatic. Every hair lost is one step closer to baldness. I could get a robe, wear a medallion and head to the airport to spread the word, whatever that is.

I have to laugh at the number of prescription bottles on my counter. I may have to start alphabetizing them. It's starting to look like my spice cabinet, which by the way, IS NOT alphabetized, so it is a total cluster. It's not good to accidentally grab Compazine instead of Claritin, just like you wouldn't want to accidentally put cinnamon in your soup instead of paprika! Is there a soup recipe with paprika?

The one thing I would be happy to get rid of is the metallic taste in my mouth from the chemo. The only thing that seems to help is chocolate. How tough is my life?? So I bought a bag of Robin's Eggs the other day (the little whoppers for Easter). I put them neatly in the pantry and Alyssa accidentally spilled the bag (half of it) on the floor. She cleaned them off the floor and Alex took the rest of the bag and said, "Mom, can I have some?" I was on the phone, so I held up my hand to show 2, thinking he would have 2 and put the bag back. The little stinker ate the WHOLE BAG and left me 2!! So now I have to hide chocolates for my chemo fix in a secret drawer! Forget getting a locked cabinet for alcohol when they are teenagers, I need the cabinet NOW for chocolate!

This week, I am hopefully going to start physical therapy for my arm. It will be nice to get some range of motion back. I haven't exercised in weeks and my "Bollywood" (hilarious belly dancing video) is waiting for my return. Alyssa and I get a total kick out of it and it really is a challenge. I have to work off all the chocolate I am eating!

I have to get busy writing thank-you notes. Everyone has been so sweet and generous. Meals, gifts, notes, thank you so much for all of them! Cindy B., that is the coolest blanket ever! Thank you so much! I cannot give thanks enough to everyone. You are all so appreciated!

I hope this note finds you all well. Keep smiling :)

Love, Connie :)

Sunday, February 15, 2009 1:25 PM, CST

I know I told you I keep all my friends who don't even know you updated on your progress as I'm sure all your other friends do as well. Anyway, my girlfriend Katie told me yesterday that you should eat with plastic silverware. When I asked her why she said people that have chemo usually have a bad metallic taste in their mouth and eating with plastic utensils curbs that...so it's worth a shot. Anyway, get your beauty sleep and make sure you take pictures! I love you, Connie.

Ellen D.

Sunday, February 15, 2009 7:20 PM, CST

Hey you! That sucks about the nausea! Make sure you tell them—they have great combos to prevent it. I have a great booklet I give to patients (made by patients) to help combat side effects. Let me know if you are interested! I miss you!!! I was so bummed to have missed the dinner. Let's catch up soon! XOXO Kristin D.

Sunday, February 15, 2009 9:17 PM, CST

Connie, you made it through!!! So sorry you were so sick though. Hopefully the meds made it a little easier. I think of you every day and look for these updates because I want to know how you are doing. I see that even a little vomit, orange pee, and chocolate missing has not taken your sense of humor. Keep smiling. Love Judy G.

I am SO TIRED. I don't have time to be tired! I have two kids who need me to be "on." I scheduled my chemo to coincide with days the kids are with their dad. By the time they return, I am feeling better. The calculated timing of poison. It's a clock with hands I don't recognize.

I try not to think of the seven remaining treatments. Eating the elephant one bite at a time has taken on new meaning. The legs are the mid-counts and the rest of the body, including the ass end, is the chemo. Big, fat and ugly. I can only think of getting to my mid-count appointment to check my white blood cell count. It is the interim week between treatments where I can expect to feel some semblance of normalcy. The few days in this journey where someone passes me mouthwash to get rid of the elephant taste.

Tuesday, February 17, 2009 6:24 PM, CST

It will be one week ago tomorrow that I had my first treatment and I feel pretty freaking fabulous. Nothing a few narcotics can't cure. So this isn't SO BAD. Tomorrow are my mid-counts—where they check my white blood cell counts. Then I will have completed "cycle one" with seven more to go. I'm still not up to snuff on all of the cancer lingo—cycles and mid-counts. If it's all the same to them, I'd rather just call it sixteen weeks of poison. Let's just call a spade a spade here.

My nose has been running like a leaky faucet in a college apartment. CONSTANT! I could just about kill myself AND my nose looks like Santa totally left me behind a couple of months ago. Who wants a cancer patient leading the sleigh anyway??

I cut my hair shorter today, inching ever closer to the dreaded bald. Next stop, Sinead. On the bright side, I am going to save HUNDREDS of dollars over the next few months on haircuts, highlighting and hair products! BONUS! I can get ready in 10 minutes and out the door I'll go! Now when Alex tells Alyssa, "You'd better stop it Alyssa, or Mom will wig out," he'll really mean it!

I have to say that this whole thing is a bit of a comic adventure. I think of that movie with Will Farrell where there is the voice-over for his every move. As I get out of bed every morning, the little voice says, "Connie is going to look at her pillow for any sign of missing hair. One hair bringing her that much closer to baldness." Followed by the crazy Jane Fonda laugh from *Monster-in-Law*. I really am going crazy, aren't I? One step away from baldness and a half step away from sucking my thumb and pissing myself while I rock back in forth in a psychiatric center. So, what brought you here? CANCER!!

Well, if you can't laugh at yourself, who can you laugh at? Everybody else I guess, but it's much more fun to laugh at yourself. So the trials and tribulations of a schizoid cancer patient continue...

Love to all, Connie

Tuesday, February 17, 2009 12:02 PM, CST

Well, it's been awhile since I've written but I read all your updates and think of you every day. It is so uplifting to know you still have your sense of humor. You crack my ass up! Every time you get sick just think of it as puking out that stinking cancer and being rid of it forever. I don't want to wait till Oct. to see you! Call me when you have time. Love you, Jen K.

Tuesday, February 17, 2009 6:34 PM, CST

God bless you is all I can say to you. I am at a loss for words at this point, more or less awestruck by your strength and courage, I am sure your two children are behind some of that...Now you never took me up on my offer. It is a standing offer. Take care stay strong and stay laughing at everyone and everything...Laura D.

PS my stepdad is still praying...

Tuesday, February 17, 2009 6:46 PM, CST

You are so brave! By reading your journal, it seems laughter is the best medicine. I think of you often and am saying prayers for you. Stay strong! I hope to see you in Plattsburgh in October!

Love, Pam H

The kids have been great! It is heartwarming when your eight-year-old daughter comes in your room to kiss you goodnight, holds your hand, and says, "Mom, you're doing great! Seven more yucky treatments left." I wonder what they are really thinking. Are they afraid I'm going to die? Or do they believe it when I tell them I will be alright?

I keep to my daily schedule to stay sane. Get the kids off to school, work, pick them up from their afterschool program, help them with their homework, make dinner and put them to bed. It's a little like Bill Murray in *Groundhog Day* with little tweaks and changes. My head is stuck in this pattern of events to keep my wits about me. The chemo and doctor visits become a part of the pattern, like the thin oval arches in a Spirograph design.

Wednesday, February 18, 2009 12:12 PM, CST

I might be feeling fabulous, but apparently I am not fabulous. My white blood cell count is half of what it should be at this point. The oncologist is concerned, but not over-the-top concerned. I have to go back and have my counts checked again on Friday morning to see if they have improved. In the meantime, I have to check my temperature often, and if it gets to 100.4 or above, they will probably hospitalize me for IV antibiotics. What a pain! If the count is still low on Friday, they may put me on oral antibiotics. Apparently, the $7000 Neulasta shot isn't all it's cracked up to be!

I am going to do my best to slow down and relax. It's a little scary to think I am so physically vulnerable. Whoever thought my life would be ruled by white blood cell counts? The kids are with their Dad until Saturday morning, so I am going to do my best to rest and get enough sleep so I am well upon their return. I will keep you all posted. Love, Connie

Wednesday, February 18, 2009 4:49 PM, CST

Dear Sweet Connie…I have been telling you to rest…you must do it…to heck with everything else…that other stuff will fall into place so don't worry about anything but yourself now. Eat your ice cream and chocolates…watch TV and rest. That is an ORDER. Love 'n stuff …Dotte C.

Wednesday, February 18, 2009 6:28 PM, CST

Connie,

Just want to let you know, although we haven't seen each other in so long, I'm thinking of you all the time and checking every day about your progress. You are the most inspiring person I know. Your attitude and outlook on all that you are going through is truly amazing!!! I'm looking forward to seeing you soon, when I come home in March. Love you lots,

Lainey H.

I guess I should be grateful to the Neulasta shot, for an opportunity to rebuild my blood cell count after the chemo killed all of my good blood cells. As a kid, I never took well to shots and this is no different. The shot itself is painful, the site sore for days. But the real clincher comes a few days later when I wake up and think I MUST have fallen asleep on the center line of a busy highway because there is no mistaking the feeling of being run over. Run over by three cement trucks all in a row with black cats hanging off the back pissing as the trucks gain momentum over my body.

The good news is, the pain eventually fades, although it takes a few days of moving VERY slowly. I am an eighty-year-old version of myself. A shot that costs seven thousand dollars? For seven grand it ought to morph me while I sleep into a perfect 10! I should wake up a blonde bombshell with a perfect size 4 body. I wake up to realize I AM a size 4, but only because my body is so wracked with poison, gaining weight is just not an option.

Friday, February 20, 2009 5:00 PM, CST

My white blood cell count has improved!! It almost doubled since Wednesday! I do have a sinus infection so I am on antibiotics AGAIN, but other than that, I am doing fairly well.

Mentally, I am always trying to find a better way to look at all of this, so today I decided to break this whole mess down into days. In 90 days, I will be done with chemo. That seemed to make it worse, so I am going back to weeks. Fifteen more weeks and I will be done with this part of the cancer journey. STILL doesn't sound any better. Well, what are you going to do? IT IS WHAT IT IS!

I have always had a theory on hair. Cut it, color it, it grows back. But when faced with the thought of not having any, the theory changes. Some people are defined by their hair. I have never been one of those chicks with a long mane of golden hair, so for me, hair is just hair. I have had it long (a long time ago), I have had it in a bob, I have had it short. I will tell you that when your hair is short, you feel totally out there. There is nothing to hide behind. It's REALLY short now, but the thought of having no hair is almost like being naked out in the middle of the street with a bunch of construction guys staring at you.

I am really struggling with knowing that within the next week, I will either be bald or pretty darn close. I have always been pretty comfortable in my own skin, but now I am going to be a skinhead. How will I feel when I look in the mirror? How will my kids feel when they see their mom with no hair? I know it is temporary and everything will be fine, but I can't help but wonder about these things. Wearing a wig just feels so unnatural. Obviously, it must be done so as to not terrify the public, but it just seems so strange.

I think the anticipation of losing my hair is actually worse than losing it. When will it all come out? Should I just shave it before I lose any? COULD SOMEONE PLEASE STOP MY MIND FROM THINKING ABOUT THE HAIR ISSUE!!!!!!!!!!

I need a drink and it's 5 o'clock HERE so it must be happy hour! Five more days until treatment number 2. Then I'll be 1/4 of the way there. That sounds better, doesn't it?? I know, I'm totally losing it.

Love, Connie :)

Friday, February 20, 2009 9:53 PM, CST

You're not losing it! (and if you were, you would be entitled to!) You actually sound fantastic. I have heard you sound much worse! :)

Hang in there. I am thinking about you!

Elena T.

Saturday, February 21, 2009 7:57 AM, CST

Connie,

I just heard of the journey you're on. Know that my thoughts and prayers are with you. I love your sense of humor. As for hair, I've always thought it was overrated. You're a beautiful person, inside and out and I don't see that changing.

Stay strong. Let me know what I can do for you.

Love,

Bev B.

Saturday, February 21, 2009 9:45 AM, CST

Hey Connie,

So glad to hear your counts have improved. Great news! I hope you've been able to rest this week. Let me know if you need anything. I could take a shot at some of those energy recipes for you. :) I understand how the prospect of losing your hair would be upsetting. I think we can all relate to that. Maybe it will help to remember that it is the chemo doing its job and getting rid of the bad cells. I have told you about my coworker. She has finished her treatment and her hair is growing back really nicely. I think she shaved hers when it started to fall out. I think you will look awesome in your wig or cool scarves in the meantime. Take care and let me know if you need anything!

Love,

Mary Beth F.

Monday, February 23, 2009 3:24 PM, CST

So there was this girl that I went to high school with and I always thought she had the most beautiful face (much like yours and I am not just saying that I am dead serious) so one day she came in and she had shaved her head and seriously she looked freaking awesome… she did it just to do it because she said her hair was taking over her face!!! I think you will look freaking fantastic. God blessed you with some damn good looks—you're lucky!

Andrea G.

Chapter 19
Hair Loss Lane

I can't believe I am obsessing over the hair situation. OK, I can BELIEVE it, but I don't WANT to. I mean, it's only hair, right? Every time I pass by a mirror, I think, "I am going to become something different than myself." But then I realize, it is only my outer self that will be different. I'll still be ME.

Years ago, in my early twenties (when I was stupid), I was engaged to this guy Mike. Turns out he was a control freak and a jerk, but I laugh at his "hair story" at my hands. I lost a bet and thinking there was NO WAY I would lose, I agreed to cut his hair in the buff. Me, not him. So I was using the clippers on the back of his head, when the attachment fell off on the floor, and OH YES, I cut straight up the back of his head right to the scalp. I yelled "Oh shit," dropped the clippers on the floor and ran into the bathroom. As I locked the door, I heard the clippers still on, vibrating against the kitchen floor.

Now it's my turn for the "Oh shit" moment, but it's not going to be just a stripe, it'll be the whole kit and caboodle.

I decide to test out the wig to calm my nerves. I go to the local grocery store in search of produce and salad dressing, but it's really an undercover mission to see if anyone notices I'm wearing a wig. I run into two people I know, and they are none the wiser. Holy crap, I might actually pull this off! And truth be told, the wig will probably fit a little better on a completely bald head. Well, one can only hope.

Tuesday, February 24, 2009 7:36 PM, CST

Well, I did it. I took control of the hair situation and buzzed it all off! The kids and I talked about it and we decided that tonight was the night. Alex chose to wait and see the end result, so that left Alyssa and I to do all the damage.

I went to my closet to get the hair clippers and started to cry. Tears were streaming down my face. I sat down on the stool in my closet and my AMAZING 8 year old daughter sat on the floor in front of me and said, "Mommy, it's going to be OK." We sat there in silence for a few minutes while I cried. I can't begin to tell you what a poignant moment that was. Just sitting there, not talking while tears streamed down my face. And she just sat there, quiet, like she understood.

So I finally got up, wiped my face and said, "I'm ready." We worked together to shave my head, laughing as we missed places, and laughing at all the hair we had to clean up. All the while, Alyssa kept saying, "Mom, you're so lucky. You won't have to blow-dry your hair anymore!" Just as we finished and were both looking at my reflection in the mirror, Alyssa said, "Well, that was a sad moment. I'm going to make you a very special dessert, Mommy." She came back upstairs with her special dessert concoction of berries, sherbet and whipped cream. Just what the doctor ordered! So we sat for awhile and ate our special dessert together. I will always remember this moment with my daughter and I think she will too.

When Alex saw the end result, he took my hand and said, "Mom, you're the best Mom ever." It is incredible to me that through this whole shit storm (and that's the best way to describe it) my children would show such amazing strength and character. We will look back at this time years from now and I will tell them what incredible kids they were throughout the whole thing.

Tomorrow, I am having my second treatment. Part of me can't wait to get it over, to know that I am 1/4 done with all of this. The other part of me is DREADING it, thinking about the nausea that is coming and the extreme fatigue. I realize that the crap part of this only lasts a few days, but just when I start to feel normal again, BAM! I have to do it all over again. I guess I will have to take one of my pre-scribed narcotics, go to bed and deal with it tomorrow. My appointment is early, so less time to think about it, which is a blessing. The mind can really mess with you. Think positive thoughts, think positive thoughts.

On the bright side, my wig fits pretty well with a clean-shaven head!

Connie :)

Tuesday, February 24, 2009 8:20 PM, CST

Connie,

Your children are your angels of mercy. They are your guidance and strength. Look, an 8 year old sitting and not saying a word is a feat in itself...she understands completely all that needs to be understood at 8. Your son, well he loves you no matter what and is so proud of you for taking the lead in this matter. Hair is only a material thing...and it does take over your life...damn...good hair days bad hair days, gone for you...yeah...no more bad ones...no waking up with hair sticking out all over and no more blow-dryers...

your daughter is right…I am so proud of your children to be so strong and supportive of you: remember, they are your strength. Love them and hug them and their strength will flow thru those hugs, kisses and tears. Hang in there, and hugs to you and the kids…love, Nancy D.

Tuesday, February 24, 2009 8:52 PM, CST

Connie,

Your daughter sounds like just what the doctor ordered. (((Hugs))) and prayers for tomorrow.

Love,

SueAnn L.

Tuesday, February 24, 2009 9:10 PM, CST

My Dear Friend, WOW!!!! What an inspiration you are to all of us!!!! You are so blessed with all the support you have, but your real strength purely comes from Alyssa and Alex. They are the reason you get out of bed in the morning. They are your future. I filled up with tears just thinking of you and Alyssa taking the big step to shave your head. Your babies are just as amazing as you…Whenever times seem tough through this journey, just think of them, think of this night and how they held your hand and guided you through. Talk to you soon, Love you, Chris F.

Tuesday, February 24, 2009 9:25 PM, CST

Connie, I am so glad that you have such great children. Your daughter understood how much you needed her and there she was, saying no words, but actually saying so much.

Hope tomorrow goes a little better than the first time. MEDICATE, SLEEP, MEDICATE and SLEEP. Thinking about you. Judy G.

Wednesday, February 25, 2009 6:39 AM, CST

It doesn't surprise me that your children are as amazing as you are. As they say, the apple doesn't fall far from the tree. Hair is nothing, love is everything...so you, my friend... have everything!

Wendy C.

Wednesday, February 25, 2009 11:16 AM, CST

I just sobbed hysterically, and not because I am sad but because I know everything is going to be alright...also because you have amazing children and as ironic as this sounds that is one of the most beautiful stories I have ever heard... you will forever be a hero to those awesome kids you have !!! I love you and them to death!

Andrea G.

Wednesday, February 25, 2009 11:40 AM, CST

Connie,

Of course your children reacted that way...you are their mother!!! Children are a reflection of their parents and you should be very proud. You're amazing, I hope I see you next week at the movies.

Love, Missy

PS Any requests? I want to bring you some food next week. xoxo

Missy T.

Wednesday, February 25, 2009 2:41 PM, CST

Connie, as I try to compose myself to type a response, I have to thank God that He has blessed you with your two wonderful children. The scripture that keeps coming to mind when I read your journal is Philippians 4:8...Fix your thoughts on what is true and honorable and right. Think about those things that are excellent and worthy of praise.

Connie, I admire your strength and sense of humor through this all. You are an amazing light to all of us that know you. May God bless you abundantly.

Lisa D.

Thursday, February 26, 2009 4:52 PM, CST

Miss Connie,

I, too, cried at your journal entry the other day about shaving your hair off, Alyssa being there with you, and what Alex said to you. Children are so wonderful, loving, caring and truly amazing in so many ways!! I continue to think about you and pray for you and your family for the strength to get through all of this. Treasure every day of your life for it is way too short!! We have to remind ourselves everyday how lucky we are to be alive, that we have a roof over our heads, food to eat, clothes to wear and the LOVE of family and friends. God bless you and your family.

Debbie D.

I will never forget what my daughter did for me that night. It was a kindness and pureness of soul I had never experienced. Later that night, after I put the kids to bed, I sat on the edge of my bed thinking, tears streaming down my cheeks. I was physically miserable, but spiritually blessed. I was dark on the outside, but there was light beaming from inside of me like a beacon. I was anxious to clear up the darkness, to beat it out of me somehow, so I could let my light shine through. Treatment #2 would lead me one step closer to the light.

Chapter 20
Round 2

Thursday, February 26, 2009 2:58 PM, CST

So I made it through chemo number 2 yesterday! 2 more of the tough ones left to go! Then 4 with Taxol and I AM DONE! I am now officially 1/4 of the way there.

I told my oncologist about the extreme nausea and the vomiting, so he put me on Emend, this $50/pill (I take 3) anti-nausea medication. I told him if it costs me $150 every treatment, I'll just throw up! My friend Rene came with me to chemo yesterday (Rene, you are such a sweetheart of a friend!). She went and picked the meds up for me and it was great that my insurance covered it with no out-of-pocket expense. Things are looking up!

I went back this morning for my shot of Neulasta and my oncologist decided to "hydrate" me with 1000 ml of fluid as well. I feel like an oompa-loompa I have so much fluid in me. So I got to sit in the chemo chair again for 2 hours today waiting for the fluid to drip ONE DRIP AT A TIME into my chest port! I told the chemo nurse today that I feel like I live at that joint!

Alyssa and I buzzed my hair just in time! It is coming out in a mad dash. I look like my brother!! (he shaves his head). We could be twins now! I'm getting used to the wig, it's not so bad. It does hurt my head after awhile and sometimes it feels like I am wearing a squirrel. I need to get used to it because I am going to be hairless for quite awhile.

I am really tired. Really, REALLY TIRED! If history repeats itself, I will be sleeping pretty much through Sunday. Take a pill, sleep. Take a pill, sleep. I'm getting the hang of this chemo thing I think. So if I don't pick up the phone or return calls for a few days, it's because I am studying the insides of my eyelids!

Many thanks for the continued thoughts and prayers, messages, gifts, food, help to appointments, picking the kids up for me (Kim and Sharon—THANKS!) and on and on. I just can't thank you all enough for everything you are doing for me. I have such AMAZING people in my life!

Love, Connie :)

Thursday, February 26, 2009 6:53 PM, CST

2 down Connie! You are amazing!!! I hope the additional meds help your stomach this time. Rest up and take care of yourself. Let me know when you are ready for the mac and cheese. I can't wait to see your wig too. I'm sure it looks adorable. See you soon.

Love,

Mary Beth F.

Thursday, February 26, 2009 10:05 PM, CST

> Hey Cons—So glad to hear you're through #2. You're going to kick ass through all 8; I know this.
>
> Your kids are incredible. Children are amazing creatures, aren't they? They don't even realize that they give us 100x more than we give them.
>
> Some sisters (including Audra and Julie) are coming into town next weekend—we'd love to come see you if you're up for it! If not, we'd totally understand. Let us know what you think—
>
> Hang tough! Love you, Kelly
>
> Kelly F.

If there is one thing I have learned in my life, and especially through this journey, it's that you have to be thankful for where you are and what blessings have been placed upon you. No matter how ugly this adventure became, I was always thankful it wasn't worse.

My friend Rene brings me to my second chemo treatment and in the waiting room, we joke about my one-titted wonderness. A woman of about sixty with big poofy hair and matching breasts sits near us. Once I am hooked up with all of my chemo accoutrement, the woman walks toward me. She says, "I didn't mean to overhear, but do you have breast cancer?"

"Yes," I said. She tells me that she has breast cancer as well, and I ask her how she is doing. She tells me that most days she has a hard time getting out of bed because she is so depressed. She was diagnosed the summer before. I assumed that she had been through all of what I was now experiencing.

She then asks me what I had done. I tell her of my mastectomies, axillary node removal, port placement, emergency surgery to remove one of my expanders, etc. I notice that one of the chemo nurses facing me listens to the conversation. The woman asks me if I have any children. I tell her yes, they are seven and eight. She asks if my husband is a big help. I tell her I am divorced. I tell her that she looks wonderful and how did she do with chemo? She says, "Oh I didn't have chemo, I just had radiation and a lumpectomy." The chemo nurse behind her rolls her eyes and I have to restrain every ounce of energy I have left not to reach out and choke her!

Here I am in the depths of HELL, let's face it. What I would give for a lumpectomy and radiation! I want to yell, "Lady, you got the freaking golden ticket of breast cancer diagnoses, and you're depressed and don't want to get up? WTF! You have YOUR hair and YOUR tits! You ought to be jumping up and down so your big ones give you black eyes! Complaining that you're too depressed to take care of your grandson during the day... I'm hoping I get to SEE grandchildren!" Someone needs to bitch-slap this woman. The chemo nurse ushers her out as she can see I'm about to blow a gasket.

Friday, February 27, 2009 3:44 PM, CST

The second treatment aftermath has been a not-so-great change from the first one. The bad part came a little sooner. Hopefully, it will go smoother from here on out. Lying in the fetal position for hours is not fun. The nausea was SO BAD last night I couldn't stand it. I am feeling a little better today. I was so sick of my hair falling out all over the place from my buzz cut, I decided to just shave it all the way today. So now I really do look like Sinead.

For all of you Facebook-ing friends of mine, I finally joined! You can spend HOURS on that site! I am not so technologically savvy, but I will get a picture on there at some point. I remember as a kid having pen pals. I guess the days of paper and ink are over!

Thanks for all of your well wishes. I will keep plugging along.

Love, Con :)

Friday, February 27, 2009 11:44 AM, CST

Hey Connie,

I want to let you know that I think of you often. Reading your journal entries is inspiring, heartbreaking, challenging, beautiful and real. It is often hard to even know what to say regarding these types of circumstances, but I can say this... for what it is worth, there is a spirit of inspiration, love, and hope that you exude. This consolation in the midst of what you are going through might not seem like much, but the power of hope and love are beyond our comprehension. Your spirit of honesty, realness, hope and love is going to get you through—for certain. Know that we think of you often, pray for you and only wish we could be closer to help. Always know you can count on us for anything if you need it.

Much Love,

Craig, Melissa and Sophia H.

Friday, February 27, 2009 4:05 PM, CST

Connie

You are 1/4 of the way done! Way to go! Keep your positive outlook. You are so brave to write so honestly on your journal site. Keep resting and take care of yourself.

Tracy L.

Friday, February 27, 2009 5:02 PM, CST

Connie—I can only reiterate what everyone else has been writing—you are such an inspiration to all of us.... . we spend sooo much time "sweating the little things in life" and through this experience with you, we realize the "little things" mean nothing...Your children are a mirror image of you...the way Alyssa was there for you during your "meltdown" and Alex being the strong little man in the background...you have done such an amazing job in raising and influencing your offspring...they are truly apples from your tree!!!! I can't wait to see you with your "temporary do"—you should have Alyssa take a picture with your phone and post it to Facebook (I am reluctant to say that I still have not posted a pic to my Facebook—will definitely take time to do that).

I, also, think of you daily and pray for you in every moment that I have a few minutes of peace each day. I feel the positive aura around you and know God's love shines down on you in a constant (Constance) ray of sunshine.

I too wish I lived closer to be able to walk through this with you...I would be holding your hand and head as you get through this nausea stage and hug you till you fell asleep.

You, my dearest friend, are the kick in the ass I need to get me out of bed and deal with my fears. I am now venturing down roads I probably would have U-turned on due to the inspiration you have provided me through your open, honest, and true-to-life communications through this difficult period of your life, and in having you in my life over the past 3 years—your energy, positive attitude and kick-ass approach have been such an triumph not only to yourself, but all of us around you.

Please call when you can, and I will call you this weekend—I love you to pieces my dear friend. Prayers, positive thoughts and energy are constant from my house to yours.

Luv ya—Kathy S.

Friday, February 27, 2009 5:33 PM, CST

Hey Connie,

I look forward to your blog. You have such a way with words. Even though I don't see you as often as I would like to, your blogging makes me feel like I am with you all the time. Keep up your fight, know we are all with you. I look forward to seeing you soon for dinner and a show.

Love ya Con!

Kellie H.

The second treatment really threw me for a loop. I was in so much pain: visceral pain, emotional pain. I sat home alone, curled up in a ball on my bed. It hurt to breathe. It hurt to think. The pain was like nothing I had ever experienced. My friend Christine brought me gingerale and I remember having to ask her to leave it on my front porch because I didn't have the strength to make it down the stairs to the front door.

Mark was off somewhere, "helping a friend," not returning my texts or calls and just plain not there for me. This journey was so very lonely. I was happy when he was around, but truth be told, it just wasn't good enough. I knew this relationship was crap. I deserved better. Whenever I gave him an out, he didn't take it, leading me to believe that this was just a bad spell in our relationship. Unfortunately, if it was a bad spell, he didn't have the fortitude to stick by me when I needed him to, only when he felt like it. Red flags lined the sky outside my house. It's a wonder I could even see the clouds beyond them.

Saturday, February 28, 2009 7:51 AM, CST

Well, another day in "Chemoville" done. Too bad it's not Margaritaville. At least I'd have a margarita! Actually, it's almost as bad as when someone dared me to eat the "worm" in college, so tequila and I aren't friends either.

I'd settle for a strawberry daiquiri with LOTS of whipped cream! AND RUM!

So the bald issue is really an adjustment. I thought it would be easier than this. It almost feels like wearing the Scarlet Letter, but instead the letter is C. Before the trip down Hair Loss Lane, no one would know I had cancer. I could stuff my surgical bra with gauze (later to find it by my abdomen, but WHO WOULD KNOW?) Now I have to wear it like a beacon, or is it a badge of honor? To be truthful, there is nothing honorable about having cancer, just the living through it part.

I am trying to wear a hat in my house at all times. For one, my head is cold. Two, I don't want to scare the Schwan's guy when he comes to the door and three, I don't want to scare myself. It's a shock when you look at yourself bald. WHO IS THAT? Oh yeah, that's ME with no hair. Soon to be no eyebrows and no eyelashes. So I throw on my $300 blonde squirrel (RIDICULOUS!) and I feel a little better.

The nausea this time has been a little better sans Thursday night in the fetal position. Now I think the ridiculously expensive Neulasta shot has kicked in, because I feel like I have been run over by a steamroller. Unfortunately, the only thing flatter on my body is my chest. Nothing a few thousand sit-ups can't match! This too shall all pass. In a few months, my plastic surgeon and I will be old buds again and I will be "reconstructed." Maybe I could get a bionic ear too, then my kids would really think, "Mom can hear EVERYTHING." They already think I have eyes on the back of my head. Now I could actually DRAW them on! That would really mess with them!

The kids are holding up really well. It's amazing to me how resilient children are. Sometimes I think they "get it" more than I do. When my Mom was diagnosed with breast cancer, I was 19. I look at Alyssa, who is 8, and think she is handling it better at 8 than I did at 19. Maybe knowing less at her age is a blessing—or so I'm hoping. And then there's Alex. At 7, he just says, "Mom, it's not like you're going to die or something." He's right. I'm not going to die. But the "something" is feeling like crap A LOT and trying not to let your kids see. It's a challenge. They know I don't feel well, and they have been total troopers.

Well, it's time for me to head the nausea off at the pass and take another Compazine. Which also means more sleep ahead. 2 down, 6 more to go. I have to keep telling myself, "YOU CAN DO THIS!"

Thank you, all of my family and friends, for seeing me through this. I will come out on the other side of this mess.

Love, Connie :)

Saturday, February 28, 2009 9:47 AM, CST

Hey there girlfriend...I will be straight and to the point... YOU NEED TO SMOKE POT!!!!!!!!!!!!! It will make things be things, and perhaps a lot more comical...Perhaps make you eat even when don't feel like eating and keep your stomach filled...I am sorry that I am unable to write more, it's end of the month in the car biz...you know how that is... Love ya girl, and light one up...Laura D.

Saturday, February 28, 2009 4:27 PM, CST

> HAHA! You are so funny, even through this tough time. I think of you every day and pray all goes well for you. Keep up your great sense of humor...it will get you through this and know that we are all thinking of you and your family!
>
> Wendy C.

Every time my mom came to see me at college, she was obsessed with cleaning. Whatever the mess, however small or large, she was on it like white on rice. One day, while cleaning the living room in the apartment I shared with a couple of sorority sisters, my mother happened upon the sacred "AD bong." My sorority bong, which had been passed down through the years to the sorority pothead who just happened to be one of my housemates. I'll never know if my mom really knew what it was. I told her it was for one of my chemistry classes. I remember calling one of my other sorority sisters to explain the unveiling. "NO SHIT!"

My mother never said a word about it.

So here I am many years later, bong-less, wondering if pot is really the answer to my continuous pain. I was never really a smoker, except the summer I stayed up at college to take graduate classes. When I held the bong on my book entitled *Substance Abuse Counseling*, I told the guys next door that I was doing research for my class. Then I would eat an entire bag of Doritos, wake up with a headache and think, what the hell did I do that for?

A friend decides to get some pot for me to see if it will help with the pain. Suffice it to say, I feel nothing, so we all know the answer to that scenario. It looks like the only break I am going to catch with this chemo is when it's all over. Not a minute sooner.

Chapter 21
Drug-Induced Comas and Other Good Times

Wednesday, March 4, 2009 1:42 PM, CST

Happy NON-CHEMO Wednesday!! I'm feeling really great today. I saw my oncologist this morning for my mid-counts, and my white blood cell counts are great. He told me my counts were so good I could go to the VA Hospital and kiss all the veterans! On the cheek of course. With masks.

So he asked me how chemo went last week. I told him that if I had been offered one of those astronaut "in case of emergency, swallow and die peacefully" pills, I would have taken one without a second thought.

"They have pills for astronauts?" he asked. Apparently he has not watched *Apollo 13*.

In the grand scheme of things, a couple of bad days is nothing, but when you are curled up in a ball it seems like an eternity.

What's the fix for next time? DRUGS! Anti-nausea, anti-anxiety (for extreme nausea) and narcotics. I asked him what I could take and when. Basically, I can take all of them at the same time! So my plan for next week is to sleep through the whole thing. Nothing like the thought of a drug-induced coma to cheer me up! I will let you know how this works out :)

I met my friend Suzanne for coffee this morning, our usual after my mid-count visit. What an amazing woman! As a cancer survivor, she is showing me the hope I need to get through this and know that I will come out on the other side. I am so grateful. It is important to look at where you are and be grateful, even when you're not in the best of places.

I am looking forward to feeling good for the next few days, spending time with Mark and the kids and just enjoying life. I keep waiting for things to be over and I realize that I need to make the most of the times I feel good in between. So we may take the kids tubing at some point this weekend. I have visions of my wig flying off and being run over. I'll have to wear a hat that ties under my chin! LOL

I hope this note finds you well. Thank you all for being so good to me.

Love, Connie :)

Wednesday, March 4, 2009 1:49 PM, CST

Applause applause…:) Way to go Connie! I'm going to write Oprah and ask her to put you on the show, but that's only with the video with you tubing with the wig and flying in the air…

Thank you again for your weekly inspirational story.

What would I do without my weekly fix?

Love you honey, Keep that chin up :)

Debra D.

Thursday, March 5, 2009 5:32 AM, CST

Connie—It is soooo GREAT to hear the smile in your update…enjoy Mark and the kids and just have fun!!!!! So the 6:00 news will have a much more lighter side than it has in the past several months…a film clip of you coming down the hill with "the squirrel" flying behind you. Ha, ha—anyway…you have come a long way and just have a short remainder to hurdle…you will do it in your "Connie style"—with flying colors.

I love you sweetie…keep positive; love, hugs and prayers from my heart to yours.

Kathy S.

Thursday, March 5, 2009 5:33 AM, CST

I'm glad to hear you're feeling well…yeah! Your sense of humor and positive attitude will see you through this. The whole tubing/wig thing sounds like *America's Funniest Home Videos*. You could be a winner! Continue to feel well. You're in my thoughts and prayers daily.

Love,

Bev B.

The thought of going tubing in theory is great. It's the thought of actually GOING that isn't so great. I lie in bed all that weekend trying to rest up. Tubing will have to wait, as will many other adventures. Suck it up sister, I think. This all will pass. Eventually.

My head runs 24/7. I don't know how I ever get any REM sleep. Seriously. Will Mark and I work out after this? Will the kids be OK with me being sick for a while longer? And when will the last of my freaking hair fall out, so I don't need to keep seeing little shaving flecks on my pillow every morning?

Thursday, March 5, 2009 11:45 AM, CST

My friend Christine pointed out to me today that I forgot to tell the "vacuum cleaner story" in my journal entry yesterday. If you need a good laugh today, this is for you.

Let me preface this by saying that those of you who know me well know that I have very little patience. OK, NO patience. I get that from my father. Sorry Dad, but you KNOW it's true :)

So the other day, I'm looking at my "almost no hair" in the mirror and getting so frustrated. If it's going to come out, COME OUT ALREADY! What is the deal? Looking at the side of my head, it was looking like cow skin with psoriasis. It was pretty ugly.

I had just finished vacuuming and I was checking out my Dyson. After all, that thing (which weighs a THOUSAND pounds) sucks up anything. Well, it's SUPPOSED to.

So I'm thinking...hmm, I wonder if I used the attachment on my head, would my hair come out? Well, OF COURSE I had to test the theory! It wouldn't be ME if I didn't, right??

I detach the tubing thing and I'm thinking...I am a total LUNATIC and if anyone could see me...OH MY GOD! You know how when the hose accidentally grabs something and it has that RAAAYYRR sound? Well, imagine that sound and my scalp being sucked into the hose. It's a clear hose, so I am witnessing the whole ordeal.

The moral of the story? The freaking Dyson DOES NOT vacuum up hair off a cancer patients head well. IF AT ALL. So I gave up and shaved my head with soap and a razor. REALLY ATTRACTIVE. What a riot.

So I'm still feeling pretty good except my nose is running like a faucet today. It's a cute look—bald with a red nose. This too shall pass.

Hope everyone is doing great today!

Love, Connie :)

Thursday, March 5, 2009 12:55 PM, CST

C you are a piece of work…you might want to write to the Dyson guy and tell him he needs to improve his vacuum cleaner…it is not doing everything it could do if properly engineered. Send him a picture. I think he would get a kick out of it. He might just invent something especially for you. What a hoot. You have made my day…Dotte C.

Thursday, March 5, 2009 4:27 PM, CST

Connie—you're too freaking funny my girl! You're just hysterical! I'm glad you're feeling better and I can't wait to see you this weekend—take care of YOU!

Julie C.

Thursday, March 5, 2009 6:55 PM, CST

You are hysterical Connie! What a sight that must have been. I really think when you are all done with this you should compile your journal into a book. You really have a way with words and the best attitude! Glad you are feeling good!

Love,

Mary Beth F.

Thursday, March 5, 2009 9:50 PM, CST

Connie, You almost made me pee my pants!!!! I could actually visualize the whole Dyson process. I am so happy you are feeling well. Keep that sense of humor. I agree…keep these journals and make a book. It is very inspirational. Love Judy G.

Friday, March 6, 2009 9:37 AM, CST

OMG!!!!!!!!!!!!!! YOU ARE TOO FREAKING FUNNY!!!!!!! Sounds like something I would do…But let me tell you…a Dyson? Get an Oreck! I love mine, if you can love your vacuum…At least I have something in my house that sucks well…Love ya…keep up the positive spirits girl, and again please dear God keep this journal and get it published!!!!!!

Laura D.

Saturday, March 7, 2009 6:42 AM, CST

OMG Connie!!!!! I am trying to type through tears streaming down my face from complete hysterical laughter with my legs crossed tightly…you, my friend are a stitch. I too can picture the whole thing as I sit here reading your journal. This will definitely be on the bestseller list this time next year. It is sooo GREAT to hear you are feeling better; I can't wait to see you. I will call this afternoon—I want to plan a road trip to Clifton Park in the next couple of weeks to see you.

Luv ya to pieces—hugs and positive energy coming your way.

Kathy S.

Tuesday, March 10, 2009 10:01 AM, CDT

Con, I was away for a few days so I just got the last update today. All I can say is that darn Dyson...it's been such a disappointment to me!

Joan F.

Wednesday, March 11, 2009 6:37 AM, CDT

Hey there Con—It was so great to see you this weekend— you look so wonderful, and you absolutely keep me in stitches. I'll be thinking of you today, and praying that it goes easier than last time. One more down! Love ya Con— talk to you soon!

Julie C.

Wednesday, March 11, 2009 11:55 AM, CDT

> Hey Cons—
>
> I just wanted you to know I was thinking about you today. May is right around the corner…
>
> Audra E.

All kidding aside, losing my hair has got to be BY FAR one of the toughest things I have ever endured. I know it seems silly. My hair is buzzed off for the most part, but it still falls out in clumps. Clumps of short hair that seem to have no end, like a dog whose shedding never seems to dissipate by brushing. I, on the other hand, would experience an end to my shedding, leaving me almost naked and stripped to a lesser version of myself.

A few days after my second treatment, I remember taking a shower. One of many, I assure you, but one that I will never forget. My hand passes over my hair with a bit of shampoo. Me, forgetting that I have very little hair to shampoo, look down at my hand after touching my head. The shock of seeing so many strands of short hair in my hand is completely devastating. I sink to the floor of the shower and sit there for what seems an eternity, crying in disbelief that this is happening to me. The water washes away the hair from my hand as I sit staring as it flows toward the drain.

It is unbelievable to think that I have to be completely broken down physically in order to rebuild myself. Who am I kidding? I was just plain ol' BROKEN. Physically, mentally, emotionally. All of it down the drain, just like my hair.

I know I laughed about it, but on the inside, I was struggling. No one really knew of my sadness because I was in "suck it up" mode and just wanted to push through. My friends though, seemed to have a pulse on my state of mind because they all rallied to my side.

A few of my sorority sisters came up to visit, and upon hearing they were coming, I had to go out to the liquor store and get some of those "test tube" shots. We had to pay homage to the past, right? So we talked and laughed and made a toast to my (almost) health. It is an afternoon I will never forget. I am so, so blessed with great people in my life. You all know who you are

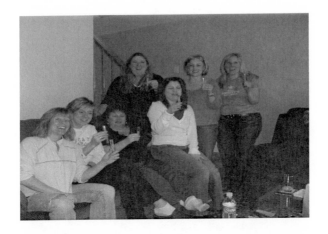

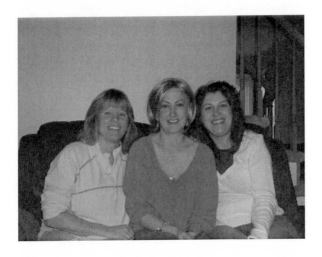

Chapter 22
Sleepless Insanity

Thursday, March 12, 2009 6:15 PM, CDT

Treatment number three is done! I am ¾ of the way through the awful chemo, then 4 more of the "not so bad" chemo treatments to go. So they are doing everything they can to help me with the nausea. They switched around the order of the chemo, giving me Cytoxan first, Adriamycin second.

They slowed the rate of the Cytoxan because it causes some nasal problems. I still had them yesterday (and still feel it). The only way I can describe it is it's like eating a roll of wintergreen Lifesavers and then going out in minus 40 degree weather and breathing in through your nose. It could be a York Peppermint Patty commercial!

I told my doctor that I haven't been sleeping, so he gave me Lunesta. Tried it out last night. Felt like I woke up in a coma and the kids ate their cereal in the dark. I felt nauseous last night and with the combination of Compazine and Lunesta, I may have beaten it.

Today, I feel pretty yucky. The nausea comes in waves and I haven't been able to eat anything. I just finished working for the day, so I am going to take a Compazine. They make me tired so I don't like to take them when I have to work.

No funny stories today. Just cannot wait to get this all over. I'm sick of being sick. Sick of not feeling like or totally being myself. I guess I can't always be a Pollyanna.

I hope everyone is doing well. Thanks for all of your good thoughts, cards and gifts. You are all so appreciated!

Love, Connie :)

Thursday, March 12, 2009 8:57 PM, CDT

I read your entries and I laugh and I cry and I laugh and I know everyone else does the same. And when you think you aren't funny the thought of even attempting to be funny with everything you're going through makes all of us just shake our heads in total disbelief. You are and should be an inspiration to all of us. And to think that you are working through all of this and still have the drive...it's amazing. I consider myself one of the fortunate few to have known you for as long as I have. Like I said to you on the phone, when I read what all of your friends do for you to assist you on a daily basis makes me sad and jealous that I can't be there for you, too. But I'm here in spirit and I know I'm lucky to have you in my life. I love you, Connie.

Ellen D.

Friday, March 13, 2009 1:29 PM, CDT

Connie...you are allowed to not be funny. I don't know how you maintain your sense of humor anyway. You are a brave soul. I mentioned to you the information I have found and will send to you. One of the things they said was to eat several "small" meals a day and eat the saltines. Stay away from spicy foods. Also, there is a nausea medicine that has a small base of POT...I will definitely highlight that baby. The weather is getting better and soon you will be able to open the windows and have the warm breeze blow in your bedroom and hear the birds singing again. I will get that information to you the first of next week. Take care my little friend...Dotte C.

Sunday, March 15, 2009 12:27 PM, CDT

Oh honey, you're SO allowed to be sick of it! I'm praying for you—if you need me you know how to find me! Thinking of you—that's one more down!!! Talk to you again soon—love you!

Julie C.

Ever since my diagnosis, sleep has proven elusive. It is a constant struggle to fall asleep and an even greater one to stay asleep. I've been trying different sleep medications, so during this chemo visit, my doctor decides to have me try Lunesta. He says he will bring the script out to me after I have my chemo.

My friend Lisa accompanies me to my treatment and the ritual begins, only this time, I have the "stuffy, by the book" nurse. She has to swab my port area with Betadine, wipe it clean and then insert the needle with my poison—and no, I don't mean a cosmopolitan. As she's doing this, she's telling me that I should take long walks during the afternoon to help me sleep at night. Are you shitting me? Lady, have you looked at me? I'm exhausted and I don't have enough energy to walk upstairs and you want me to take a walk? How about you take a walk, AWAY from me, before I lose my shit! How about that? She drips the Betadine down my chest, so I grab a cotton swab to clean it off and she totally freaks out and says she has to start over because my heart could become infected if the area is not completely sterile. I say, "Just do it, I'll take my chances."

I look over at Lisa and I can tell she sees I'm edging very close to the abyss of freaking out on this chick. The nurse gets so flustered that she has another nurse come over to finish my chemo. This is the one and only time during my poison reign that I come so close to going postal.

I'm going to come clean. That was the start of a bad week for me, and I was a totally pissy person. I'm really not one to turn inward, but at this particular point in the journey, I was making the sharp right turn to Pity City. No long stretches of road with street lights, just a couple of stop signs like the small town I grew up in— where everyone knew everyone else's business. A great place to raise small children, and yet so tiny, a teenager had the most miniscule span of wiggle room to spread his or her wings. A beautiful place, but one where living under a microscope of sorts became commonplace. Now the microscope was held by my doctors, not my neighbors.

Finally, my chemo is finished and my doctor brings out my script. Sleep is going to happen this night, for sure! I make a mental note to request my favorite nurses for future poisonous visits.

Chapter 23
The Blue Hat

Tuesday, March 17, 2009 3:19 AM, CDT

Happy St. Patrick's Day everybody! Today, my mother, God rest her soul, would have been 66. She was the most amazingly funny, caring, giving person you could ever know. What has been so scary to me through all of this, is knowing that I am fighting the very fight she was unable to win.

As I have been going through my own HELL, and it is hell, I have been thinking a lot about my mom and how she must have felt. Her cancer was never a topic of conversation. It was the pink elephant in the room. She was so completely private about her journey. She was an incredibly strong woman and I always have admired her for that. For me, reaching out to my friends and family and laughing as best I can at all of this, is my way of coping, and I thank you all for being a part of that.

So many times going through this I wish I could just tell her, "I know how you were feeling. I know what you were thinking." I wish I could reach back in time and tell her that I understand. Sometimes, I feel like this little "adventure" is a torturous journey of the MIND and the body.

Mostly when I think about my mother, I have something to laugh about. It seems we were always laughing about something. Some crazy thing she did (usually to embarrass us, but not on purpose!). My kids and I always seem to be laughing about something too.

When I got my wig, Mark had me try on this poofy blue hat. Alyssa was with us and gave me the "Are you kidding me Mom?" look. The lady at the wig place threw it in, kind of like when you buy a car and they throw in an extra set of keys or a stripe on the side.

A couple of nights ago, the kids helped me try on scarves. Let me tell you, I looked like a complete spaz trying to tie those scarves on my head and most of them made me look like I needed a dot on my forehead (don't mean to offend, but seriously!).

So Alyssa says, "Mom, where's that ugly blue hat?" She takes it out of my closet and stuffs all of her hair in it and prances around my room. It was HILARIOUS! It has this whacked-out flower thing on the side of it that is as big as her cheek! She gets my camera and says, "Mom, take a picture!" Well, this leads to Alex trying on the hat, which, with his boy pajamas on, added a whole new level of hilarity! The three of us were laughing so hard, we were howling! Now all three of us have a picture of ourselves wearing the ugly blue hat and a very comical memory!

So we finish cracking up about it and I say to Alyssa (kidding), "If you don't behave, I'm going to pick you up from Y-time (their after school program) wearing the blue hat."

She says, "Mom, I would DIE. I would NEVER be able to show my face again!" This little exchange reminds me so much of myself with my mother. I can't believe at her age of 8, I am already on my way to embarrassing her .

So I pick them up at Y-time the next day and Alyssa asks me, "So Mom, where's the blue hat?"

I say, "I have spared you a day of humiliation." She raises her eyebrow at me as if in a dare, and I will tell you, IT IS ON! I am going to wear that blue hat to pick her up! I've turned into my mother! And for that, and all I am going through, I just laugh and laugh.

My mother, wherever she is, is laughing and saying, "You get back what you dish out kid." I guess I deserve it. But I might as well have as much fun with it as if I can, right??

I feel much better. This last chemo was tough, as are ALL of them, but I am almost at the halfway point, which is keeping me somewhat sane (if that is at all possible). Alyssa told me the other night, "Mom you have 5 more treatments. 10 more weeks of the yucky stuff." I guess when your 8-year-old can look at it like that, you have to as well. I will get there.

I hope this notes finds you all well and that you enjoy your St. Patrick's Day. The kids want me to put green food coloring in their milk this morning to make their *Kix* green. Should make for an interesting conversation with the school counselor or nurse later. I could top it off by having one of them wear the blue hat!!

Go have a laugh today and find your own blue hat (or green if the spirit moves you)! I'm going to pick my children up today and embarrass them!! Maybe.

Love, Connie :)

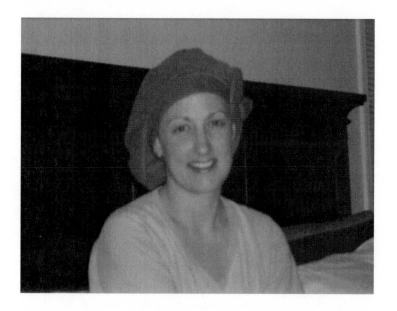

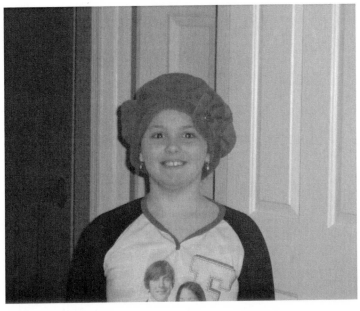

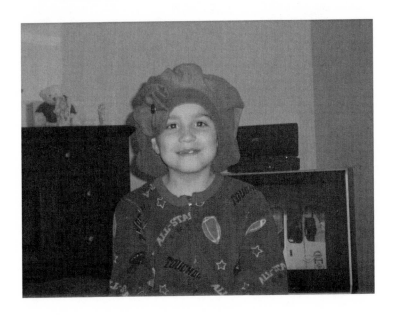

Tuesday, March 17, 2009 7:36 AM, CDT

Con—Your Mom is smiling down on you today with pride and admiration. You are such an amazing woman with a spirit that rises above all else. You have only a few more months of this and we are all here to get you through it. I, as well as many, many others who have shared this journal with you, love you like a sister and we are all here to make this horrible journey together and, my dear friend, there is a "pot of gold" at the end of the road. You will be healthy and free of this awful disease, and be able to enjoy your life, your children and your friends. You hang in there sweetie; my prayers, positive energy and love are with you each and every day. Happy St. Pattie's Day, and Happy Birthday Mom!

Kathy S.

Tuesday, March 17, 2009 9:32 AM, CDT

Yo Cone,

Happy St Pat's Day. Even though I'm half Italian I still celebrate with a few Guinnesses. Anyway, glad to see you are staying strong. That was a good testament to your mother—so much of her is in you and that's a good thing! She was an amazing woman and I miss the times we had at your house. (I think she liked calling me Juan too!)

I just happened to look at the number of visits on this site. 2185 currently—man, that's a lot of your peeps wanting to check in to see how you are doing.

Keep strong and always let me know if you need a Pizza Hut delivery...

Love ya!

Juan (John P.)

Connie,

Happy St. Patrick's Day to you too, and Happy Birthday Mom!!!!

Your mom knows what a courageous daughter she has, and she knows that you are going thru exactly what she went thru...not what she had planned for her daughter, but she brought you up strong, and she knows you can beat this damn thing. She is egging you on to do your silly antics with the kids, and to make them laugh as they make you laugh. They want you to greet them at aftercare with that hat...no doubt in my mind. They are proud of you...they are proud of how you are handling all this...and they love you to the moon and back...

Your writing today was a wonderful tribute to your Mom... she was a special person for sure.

Love ya,

Nancy D.

Connie...HAPPY ST. PATRICKS DAY! You are just too funny...your sense of humor is abundant and it sounds like your daughter is not far behind...that old saying "the apple doesn't fall far from the tree" seems to be fitting. It is nice that you think about your mom and some good times. She may be around you right now and that is why your thoughts about her are so strong. The weather is beautiful today...I hope you were able to go outside and enjoy the sun. I am planning to send you the information I have been talking about tomorrow. I have to finish highlighting important parts. Are you having corned beef and cabbage tonight? I am dying for some of it. There is a restaurant here in Bolton Landing serving it tonight. I may go down and have some. I really enjoyed your message today...it lifted me...I have had a crazy day...too involved to repeat...nothing bad...just a comedy of errors. Oh well, that's the way things go...Lots of love to you my friend...Dotte C.

Wednesday, March 18, 2009 10:10 AM, CDT

Connie, I too remember my mom through your emails and trials and tribulations. It will be 20 years this August since her passing and it's still like yesterday. Your mom knows your feelings every step of the way: the good ones and the bad ones. Funny thing happened a few weeks back. I went to a psychic. Yeah whatever, it was for entertainment purposes only. After speaking about a lot of nothing, the lady said she has a strong feeling from someone who has passed and she got up and asked me to stand and she said I am going to hug you because your mom thinks you need a hug from her...OK so I kind of felt freaky but here is why I am telling you this...The thing I miss the most from my mom is the hugs...the good-time hugs, the bad-time hugs and the just-for-the-sake-of-a-hug hugs...and she knew that. Twenty years later she still knew what I needed. So somewhere up there, your mom knows what you are going through and what you need. Just believe that they may not be here for us to have physical touch, but they are in our hearts to give us the soul connection and the heartfelt touch…Stay happy and hug yourself today: it's from your mom…love ya

Laura D.

My father often refers to my mother as "an angel on earth," and that is exactly what she was. She had a remarkable way of putting everyone at ease and pointing out the good in every situation. Since her passing, I have often thought, "What would my mother think about…" when I was faced with a decision. I remember the day of my diagnosis. The shock of finally knowing the day had arrived, however morbid it was of me to have expected it. I remember thinking, "I will deal with this head-on, grab it by the balls, and crush it." There are moments when you are faced with a fork in the road. One direction leads you down a path of misery and self destruction, the other one passes through misery, but you know it will eventually turn into a brighter place. I decided early on which fork in the road I was going to take. Obviously, it was going to be the one with the brighter place at the end.

It wasn't all about ME. It was about the two kids who sat in the backseat along the journey. I couldn't take them to an ugly place and tell them, "Oh yeah, I forgot to tell you, where we end up is going to be REALLY ugly." My kids could have their heads buried in their Game Boys and DSI's for the crappy part of the ride, but at some point, they would have to look out the window at the beautiful view. I tried my best to get them to laugh and talk about the ugly parts as the brighter place edged closer into view.

Thursday, March 19, 2009 9:57 AM, CDT

Hey everyone! So many of you have called and emailed me asking me if I wore the blue hat. Of course I did!! I showed up at their afterschool program on Wednesday wearing the ugly blue hat. Alyssa's eyes almost popped out of their sockets and Alex just laughed. We all have to lighten up, right?

So I just got back from having my mid-counts done. My oncologist is on vacation, so I had the pleasure of seeing the gloom-and-doom oncologist in the office. He would make a great funeral director, especially since every time I have to see him I wonder if I need to head to the nearest funeral home to make my arrangements.

"I'm concerned because your WBC is on the low side."

To which I respond with, "Well, I'm on an antibiotic, so that should kill everything that ails me." (Not to mention the big-ass glass of wine I had last night followed by 3 cosmo-politans!!! LOL!). I neglect to tell him this last part for fear he will pass out.

All the while he is talking, I can't stop looking at the hair growing out of his ear. What is it with men and ear hair?? I don't get it. I have to bite my tongue to keep from saying, "Dude, buy yourself some clippers and go to town on the ferret you've got coming out of the side of your head."

Despite my "near death's door" blood count, I am feeling pretty well. MANY thanks to my friend Deana for taking me out last night. I almost feel human again. There's nothing a few cocktails can't help!

I hope you are all doing well. I am looking forward to spring on Friday, which will also mark the 2 month countdown to my being finished with chemo. I'm trying to just focus on the finish line!

As always, thanks for the cards, well wishes, and most importantly, COCKTAILS!!

Love, Connie :)

Thursday, March 19, 2009 9:35 AM, CDT

Hey sweets,

As always, you managed to crack me up. It was sooo great seeing you! We have to make a date for cocktails more often so you can enjoy your week off and feel like a human hottie again, and may I say you are most certainly still a hottie. Even with your wig off, you are truly beautiful. Why can't Sinead O'Connor bring back the trend? You would rock it girl!

Love ,

Deana L.

Thursday, March 19, 2009 9:46 AM, CDT

You're continuing to rock this thing! Ken and I look forward to each of your journal entries—they often leave us ROFL. You've got a way with words and are just too funny. Good for you—laughter IS the best medicine. I indulged many good thoughts about Jackie (*my mom*) on Tuesday, which was my birthday too. She was just about the first person to warmly welcome me into the family, and I'll always be grateful.

Keep up the great work!

Kathryn G.

Thursday, March 19, 2009 10:12 AM, CDT

Hi Connie!

Your sense of humor is as great as ever! This definitely needs to be published when you are done. Perfect memoir. Thank you for all of your updates. I wish I could come visit you, but soon! I will be coordinating with my driving partner on some dates. My thoughts and prayers are always with you. Thanks for the laughs!

Love,

Britt B.

Thursday, March 19, 2009 11:40 AM, CDT

You are such a riot, Connie! Your story about the ear hair reminds me of the *Brady Bunch* episode where Greg visualizes the guy administering the driver test in his underwear to deal with his nervousness. But you may not be old enough to remember that one. I'm sorry I missed the cosmos. Count me in next time! What a beautiful tribute to your mom. I'm sure she is watching over you as your guardian angel with so much love and pride for your courage and positive attitude in dealing with all of this. So glad that you are in the homestretch. See you soon!

Love,

Mary Beth F.

Thursday, March 19, 2009 12:40 PM, CDT

Fabulous seeing you last weekend—or was it 2 weeks ago?! You look amazing—and the wig is gorgeous. It truly amazes me how positive and optimistic you remain. I have a lot of patients I am managing right now with breast cancer and they would benefit SO MUCH from your knowledge and support! Have you ever considered a career change????? Have a great day!!!!

xoxoxoxo—Kristin D.

Thursday, March 19, 2009 3:54 PM, CHey Connie,

Your blue hat story made me laugh and cry—quite an accomplishment! You should really consider putting your entries together and sending them to a publishing house. They are so real and inspirational! Hope you are doing well. Sorry I couldn't visit with the other ADs a couple of weeks ago—I would have loved to see you and wish you well in person. Stay strong!

Tracy L.

Wednesday, March 25, 2009 4:15 PM, CDT

Hi Con - Just wanted you to know I'm thinking of you today—one more down! Loved the blue hat story, and the tribute to your mom was beautiful. Take care—my prayers and good vibes are with you! Love ya—Jules

Julie C.

Chapter 24
Halfway There

I used to DREAD going to the oncologist for my mid-counts. For one, I was sick of the drive there. Second, it was like checking in with Dr. Death every other week. My health tied into a number driven by white blood cells. The announcement of the count was preceded with, "How are you feeling?"

If I could depart from niceties, I would say, "How the hell do you think I feel? I've been poisoned as if attacked by venomous snakes and then had to spend time doing second and third grade homework!" OK, I may have actually said this once or twice. But the one positive feature of being sick is that you get a few free passes for bitchiness.

Sunday, March 29, 2009 10:46 AM, EDT

I survived my fourth and final A-C treatment on Thursday! Whoohoo! Now I am halfway through chemo! Thank goodness I am finally turning the corner. I'm still feeling a bit tired and rundown from this last treatment, but overall, I am just so happy that it is over with. From what I hear from other patients and the nurses in my oncology office, the last four treatments of Taxol should be a breeze compared to what I have been through.

The Taxol will not come with the extreme nausea of the A-C, but it comes with other side effects. I asked my oncologist on Thursday what I have to look forward to with these next four treatments, and apparently allergic reaction to the chemo is a (rare) possibility, along with anaphylactic shock (oh JOY!), but most common is numbness in the fingers and toes. They monitor this all very closely, so I'm not too worried about it. What's another poisonous cocktail at this point? Bring it on.

My poor oncologist. This past week I was in one of my "I'm going to ask him a million questions" moods. I asked him when I would be getting my chemo port out. In case you don't know what this is, it is a plastic thing that is hooked up to one of my veins right under my skin below my clavicle. It is ANNOYING and UNCOMFORTABLE and I want it out ASAP. I'm thinking since I am in the home stretch, I want to know when I'm going to get my expander back in on my right side and when this port is coming out. So of course, I ASK.

His answer? "I'd like to keep the port in for a year."

My response??? "ARE YOU ON CRACK? This thing is coming out as soon as my blood count is good enough for surgery." He would like to keep it in just in case of a reoccurrence. I don't want to even think about that, and if it does happen, I'll have another one put in. The mission here is "How Connie got her boobs back," NOT "How Connie had to live with an annoying port in her chest for a year in case her cancer came back." So the long and the short of it is, it's coming out as soon as possible! I want to get back to normal as soon as possible.

I am so grateful for the support you all have given me: the calls from friends from ALL OVER and forever ago! How great it has been to reconnect with so many! It just makes me realize that EVERY friendship you have in your life is meaningful.

Alyssa and Alex have been the most incredibly supportive children I could have ever imagined. I know this has been difficult for them, but they have been troopers, and in the midst of it all, my biggest cheerleaders. They are reading a book right now that my friend Sue lent us called, "*The Year My Mother Was Bald.*" I'm living with the baldness, but I know that having a bald Mom has been tough on them too. They are remarkable children and I am so very proud. And BLESSED. Truly blessed.

I am also very blessed to have a wonderful man in my life who sees me for me even when I am sick, bald and definitely not myself. What a remarkable human being to stand by me through all of this difficulty I am facing. To find ways to make me laugh when it's the last thing I feel like doing (but really need), holding my hand when I am feeling so nauseous I could just die, making me eat when it's the last thing I want to do (but really need), caring about me like no one else ever has. For this and so much more, I am eternally grateful for his love and support. Mark, you are an incredible man to stand by me and love me through all of this. I love you so very much.

Thank you all so much for your continued thoughts and prayers! I'm half way there!

Love, Connie :)

Sunday, March 29, 2009 11:11 AM, EDT

Hi Connie: Just checking in to give you my positive thoughts and encouragement. You are doing great, you are truly a warrior, you are setting a great example for your children, you are going to be better just around the corner, you have a huge amount of good people around you. Don't ever give up, keep moving forward. Thoughts and prayers, Jonathan K.

Sunday, March 29, 2009 7:08 PM, CDT

Miss Connie, Congrats on being halfway there!! Keep up your good spirits. I am so glad you have a good man in your life to help you through your adventure. I too have been blessed with a good man, finally. I think about you often and am so glad to hear your children are supportive and you are all doing OK.

Take care and God bless.

Debbie D.

Sunday, March 29, 2009 9:09 PM, CDT

Dear Connie,

I am so glad you have this site so I can read all your updates. You are a blessing to so many. To hear about all you are going through and will come through is a testimony to the power of supportive friends, and your positive attitude with loving family. I hope to meet Mark one day. What a remarkable man! You are in my thoughts and prayers.

Maureen L.

Monday, March 30, 2009 7:57 AM, EDT

I'm so glad to hear that you are halfway. The second half will be a lot better than the first half. That makes me smile to hear about Mark being there for you—that is what you deserve. You're an amazing woman!!

Love, Kate D.

I had never really mentioned Mark in my journal before. He read it once in a while and asked me why I never mentioned him in my writing. Truth be told, I didn't mention him because I was never sure if he was IN my life. I always felt like an extra on the *Mark Show*. My appearances were determined by his mood. I was grateful for the times he was there for me, but his absences often felt like another round of chemo. Maybe writing about him made the relationship we once had seem more of a present situation. Reading everyone's comments about how great my relationship with Mark was made me sick to my stomach because deep down, I knew the truth. It was a façade. A façade that good health would either make real or be the last brick to remove before the fall.

Friday, April 3, 2009 2:36 PM, EDT

49 more days and I will be done with chemo! Thank God because I am tired of feeling like something the cat dragged in. Actually, dragged, run-over, stomped on, peed on and then run-over again. THAT WOULD BE MOST ACCURATE.

I have been sick with a chest cold that I can't seem to kick and I am on some heavy duty antibiotics for 21 days. If I am not better by next week, I may not get my chemo. Which, mentally, could be my doom. Counting down the days is what is keeping my sanity.

The kids had a blast the other night wearing my wig. What a couple of freaks they were: laughing, tossing the hair around and saying, "Hi, I'm Connie." It was hilarious. Thank God they are such great sports about this!

You all know that I am a total spaz. I am going to attempt to put the blue hat pictures on the site so you can all laugh at what lunatics we look like. I hope you all laugh as much as we have about the blue hat. I also have a couple of pictures with my wig.

I hope you are all doing great! Thank you so much for all of the beautiful cards. They so keep my spirits up!

Love, Connie :)

Tuesday, March 31, 2009 12:55 PM, CDT

Hello Doll,

Well once again I can see that you do still find the humor in all of this. It's wonderful for you that you have a good man to stand with you and that your children have been what they need to be…the children they are.

I am glad that you are over what seems to be the yucky part and now hopefully will be downhill from here.

Love and prayers and hugs to you. Take care. Laura D.

Friday, April 3, 2009 5:05 PM, EDT

Hey Girlfriend!!!!! LOVE THE PICS! That Blue Hat beats all!!!!!!!!!!!!!!! What an amazingly beautiful family you have—thanks so much for sharing the photos; it makes me feel a little less far away.

You are on the homeward stretch now honey, so just keep those feet planted and your mind and spirit in the right mode and you will do just amazingly. I know you are experiencing a lot of scary things right now, but your attitude and spirit are in the right place.

I love you and the prayers, positive energy and karma all continue to come your way each day—from my heart to yours.

Love ya—Kathy S.

Friday, April 3, 2009 8:09 PM, CDT

Connie,

Thank you for the pictures…they are priceless.

Take care of that cold as I know you will. Things are going to be OK.

Just think of all the things you have to be thankful for your 2 beautiful children, Mark, your beautiful blue hat, your beautiful wig, your sense of humor and all your positive friends rooting for you on this journey. You can do it. If anyone can, you can.

You have inspired me beyond belief with your antics and wonderful writings.

Love Nancy D.

Friday, April 3, 2009 8:18 PM, CDT

Connie, Your blue hat is THE BOMB. Too cute, yet too funny. I am counting down your days with you. Take care of that cold. The pictures with the sisters made me wish I had been able to join you all. But as you know it was best for you I didn't as I ended up with pneumonia. It was someone watching out for you. Keep the faith. We all think of you every day. 1/2 way there!!! Love, Judy G.

Chapter 25
Sick and Tired

I was so sick at this point in the journey. Really, I could barely breathe. I knew that Prednisone was what I needed to take to come out of it, but it was just not an option, because it would weaken my ability to fight off infection even further. I was scared. It was one thing to have foreign poisons enter my body to fight off what I couldn't see, it was quite another to have the feeling that my own body had turned against me.

I was so beaten down. I had another occupant living with me, the elephant that was sitting on my chest, choking me and flattening my spirit. The fat bastard. If it would just get the hell off, I would feel better. My head kept going to a bad place where the end of chemo was miles and miles away and my own demise, just around the corner.

The nurse practitioner at the oncologist's office had told me that this halfway point was really difficult for so many people. "Why," I thought? "I'm halfway done!" I've always been the-glass-is-half-full kind of person, so at this point I was happy that it was actually half empty. The nurse told me that it was the point at which people are happy they have finished the first half, but often are defeated at the thought that they are only halfway done. Well that was an uplifting visit, I thought to myself as I choked on my own phlegm leaving the office.

Friday, April 10, 2009 8:44 AM, CDT

Well, I made it through my 5th treatment yesterday! 3 more to go and I will be done with all of this madness! I feel good so far, just very tired and my body aches like I ran a marathon. All of you who know me KNOW that I have no idea what that feels like, but let's just pretend.

I have to thank my friend Chris H. for coming with me to a taxing 5 hour appointment. No pun intended (I received Taxol at the appointment). The thing I was most worried about yesterday was having an allergic reaction to the chemo, and the poor woman sitting next to me had a reaction to hers. This is really scary stuff.

I FINALLY turned the corner. 41 days from today is my last treatment. It's hard to believe it's been 5 months since I was diagnosed. A lot has happened in those 5 months.

Today is the 13-year anniversary of my mother's death. Some days it seems like forever ago and other days it seems just like yesterday. Every day I hope that I am half the woman and mother that she was. She was such an incredible person. I know she would be sick to know what I am going through. I really wish I could tell her that I understand. All the days she must have felt horrible and still did all the things she did, I don't know how she ever did it.

The physical part of this is awful, I am not going to lie. Awful, but livable. It is the mental side that is a struggle some days. You don't realize when you are healthy how quickly things can change. The stupid things you complain about really don't matter when you are curled up in a ball from chemo and just wish it would be over already. Now that I know what a REALLY BAD day is, I am so looking forward to some great days! And they are just around the corner.

The kids are doing great. We have been playing a card game as a countdown to the end of my chemo. We have assigned all of the face cards a value. For example, when we pull a King, we order a pizza. And each day we rip up a card as we get closer to the end. I owe them 2 trips to the dollar store because they pulled a Queen 2 days in a row. The little stinkers remember EVERYTHING!

I hope you all have a wonderful Easter. The kids are with their Dad and I will be spending the holiday with Mark. I am looking forward to a quiet holiday and getting rested up.

Much love to all, Connie :)

Friday, April 10, 2009 2:45 PM, CDT

My dearest Connie!!! You are almost THERE!!!!!!!!!!!!!!!!!
It does seem pretty incredible that the time has gone by like it has...I'm sure there have been days for you that it doesn't seem to move at all.

I just got back from Good Friday services—lit a candle for both you and your Mom—prayers and tears pouring out of me at the same time. You are soooo precious to all of us, and what a journey you have had to endure—but you have...and that, my dearest friend, is the most important thing of all.

Your mother has been right beside you giving you that extra push when you've needed it, a cool hand to your forehead and your amazing ability to keep it all together.

I hope your time this weekend with Mark is restful. I will try to call you on Saturday to check in. You are surrounded by so many people who love you and cherish your friendship. Keep positive thoughts; my prayers, positive energy and hugs…from my heart to yours,

luv ya—Kathy S.

Friday, April 10, 2009 3:07 PM, CDT

I love the pictures—especially the blue hat ones! You are in the homestretch. Do what you need to for yourself. I hope you can rest and relax this weekend. If you have chance, check out the comedian Jim Gaffigan on Comedy Central— he is hilarious. Happy Easter and I'll talk to you next week!

Love,

Mary Beth F.

Saturday, April 11, 2009 9:52 AM, CDT

Happy Easter—Connie

Call me next week!!! The finish line is getting within reach!!!!

Rene S.

Monday, April 13, 2009 6:04 AM, CDT

Connie,

I hope you got the rest you were looking forward to and had a great Easter. Love the blue hat pics :)

You are such an inspiration!   You're a strong person. Your strength and faith will see you through this.

Looking forward to seeing you soon. :) Take good care of yourself and know my thoughts and prayers are with you.

Love ,

Bev B.

I remember sitting in the chemo chair, all of the old people in recliners next to me hooked up to their very own poison. I held my breath and waited for the liquid venom to enter my veins. My greatest fear with this change of chemotherapy was an allergic reaction. Just as I'm thinking, "I'm in the clear," the woman next to me had an anaphylactic shock reaction to the same chemo I was receiving. HOLY SHIT! I will say again, HOLY SHIT! The nurses scrambled to shut off her IV and give her oxygen. Unbelievable. I held my breath, waiting for my own reaction.

Let's face it. If I held my breath even ONCE while waiting for all of the bad shit to pass, I would have turned blue long ago and keeled over dead. Thank god I know how to breathe. I have found myself in many a situation where breathing has been my only salvation.

There were days when slapping my wig on was like throwing on a furry hat, and others when I actually felt fan-freaking-tastic. With my wig and some makeup, I sometimes felt nearly human. Long before I was sick, Mark bought me these pretty cool sunglasses for riding on the back of his motorcycle. The one clincher (no pun intended) was that they were so tight on my head I needed a couple of Excedrin.

During one of my looking and feeling fabulous episodes, I had one of those Excedrin moments with the sunglasses while sitting in my car at a major intersection in my town. As I removed the sunglasses, my wig turned completely sideways on my head. I thought nothing of it as I adjusted it back to normal, and as I looked back to the road, this guy on the other side of the intersection looked at me with his head cocked to one side with a WTF look on his face. I put my sunglasses back on, looked over at him, and gave him the thumbs up sign. What are ya gonna to do? I could have really scared the shit out of him and taken the wig off completely!

Chapter 26
Shin Splints and Psychosis

Tuesday, April 14, 2009 8:16 PM, CDT

38 days until my last chemo treatment! This first Taxol treatment seemed to go well in the beginning. I felt great! I had dinner at a friend's house the night after (along with a couple of cocktails, of course!), felt great and thought "This is going to be a breeze."

2 days after my treatment, I have this horrible leg pain. Like having shin splints times 10 ALL DAY LONG! It is so strange, because the pain goes from my knees to my feet on both legs, not just one. It got so bad today that I went to see the doctor. I saw an oncologist in the practice (not mine) and he said that the pain is due to nerve damage from the Taxol—it is not typical, and often affects his young, healthy patients. Basically, he told me the old ladies don't even notice! LOL!

I will be seeing my oncologist on Thursday and because of the leg situation, he may either change my chemo, or bring the dosage down. Or who knows? He could say, "This poor girl has been through enough. Let's call it a day." I know, wishful thinking. The doctor told me today that the nerve damage can be permanent/semi-permanent, or take months to go away. On a much smaller level, I now know how it must feel to have chronic pain, even if it's just for a few days (it's enough!). I can't even imagine having to deal with this pain on a daily basis. The narcotics they have given me aren't even touching the pain. A few more days of this and you'll probably find me rocking in a corner, drooling all over myself.

I JUST WANT TO FEEL NORMAL!!! I want to feel normal, I want to look normal. I JUST WANT TO BE NORMAL!! I know, my "normal" is completely spastic, but it's still MY normal!

I had to laugh tonight because the kids and I went out to dinner and when I sat down, I almost took my wig off. It was hot and it felt like a hat, so what the heck? How is it that your own hair doesn't feel like a hat? The waitress at Friday's almost had a bald chick to wait on tonight!

My friend Suzanne gave me the Melissa Etheridge CD with the song "I Run For Life" on it, which if you don't know, is a beautiful song about running for all of us with breast cancer. The kids listened to it and I said nothing about what the song meant, and Alyssa said, "Mom, that song makes me cry." It was so great that she got it. These kids are so smart; much smarter than we can ever give them credit for being. I remember hearing the song when it first came out, thinking about my mother and thinking that no amount of running would ever bring her back. Now I listen to that song and think about running for myself and running for Alyssa and everyone else in my life that is (or will be) affected by breast cancer. So the kids and I have decided that we are going to put a team together for the breast cancer run in October. We are going to get special t-shirts made up and get all of our friends (yeah, YOU!) to run or walk with us, FOR HOPE. Hope for a healthy future, because that is what we have been focusing on.

I hope this note finds you all well. Happy and HEALTHY. Thank you for all of the beautiful cards. They SO lift my spirits. I have amazing friends and am so blessed! Thank you all!

Love, Connie :)

Thursday, April 16, 2009 9:12 PM, CDT

Hey Connie,

I'm so sorry you're having leg pain. It must be tough! You're in my thoughts and prayers. Here's hoping you can stay on schedule and have this over with soon!

Tracy L.

Someone beat the shit out of my legs while I slept. Either that, or I ran a marathon in my sleep trying to escape the grips of Freddie Krueger. I cannot believe the leg pain.

I would say that I am a person who has a very high tolerance for pain. I mean, I endured years of a not-so-happy marriage, so a little leg pain is doable, right? I should have allowed Freddie to get me and drag me to the depths of hell because, well, I was already there. I lay in bed, miserable and in pain, thinking of all our military veterans. So many of whom have experienced life-changing injuries, to ensure that I was able to live in a country where treatment for my illness would even be possible. I wondered how many were lying in their beds at that moment in pain. Thousands, maybe millions, I didn't know.

It is then that I realize that no matter what is dished out to me, I will take it and deal. It is not my choice to deal with it, it is my obligation.

Thursday, April 16, 2009 5:55 PM, CDT

I went to the oncologist today for my mid-counts. My blood levels are OK, but I am experiencing neuropathy in my legs which is unusual (figures!). My oncologist gave me some medicine to try to help with the pain, as it is not subsiding AT ALL. He said that joint pain is common with the Taxol, but not what I am experiencing.

He wants me to come back next Tuesday to reassess the situation. If the pain has not subsided, he may change my chemo treatment for Thursday. He said he is hoping to keep me on the Taxol because that is my best chance for a cure.

I am in a lot of pain and I am hoping this medicine will work! I'll keep you all posted.

Love, Connie :)

Friday, April 17, 2009 7:14 AM, CDT

Karlie said this to me last night: "Friendship is like peeing on yourself. Everyone can see it but only you can feel it." Let's promise to pee on each other forever. I love you Bramer and pray for you to have peace and continued strength. xoxo, Laurie K.

Friday, April 17, 2009 9:35 AM, CDT

Thinking of you Connie!!! Hope you feel better soon…

Love,

Wendy C.

Monday, April 20, 2009 9:44 AM, CDT

Thinking of you and hoping you are feeling better. Can't wait to see you!

Joan F.

Monday, April 20, 2009 11:24 AM, CDT

Hey girl!! Sorry to hear of your pain. This too shall pass. I will run in the breast cancer thingy...just let me know!! Think of you often. Love, Jen K.

Monday, April 20, 2009 5:37 PM, EDT

Hey Cone!

You are doing great. I am so proud of you!!! Your outlook and attitude have been and remain awesome! We all love and admire you big time!

See you next month!

Love Kurt, Melissa, Jake & Madie Mooooooo!

Tuesday, April 21, 2009 4:51 PM, CDT

Hi Connie,

I just got caught up on your journal as I have been away and out of touch...but am back home now.

You are right...the blue hat is pretty bad! Everyone looks the same in it!

You might be wondering like the rest of us why more set-backs? Doesn't this seem like enough already? Only God knows the answer to that but we will be faithful and keep praying…as that is exactly what HE wants us to do, so hang in there and know you are loved, cherished, treasured, and you can only be stronger through it all! Love you…Anna B.

I remember feeling as if I had been struck by lightning when my doctor told me that my chemo regimen was my best chance at a cure. The thought that cancer could or even would have the balls to linger completely scared me to death. It was the moment I realized I would have to worry about this for the rest of my life. What I really wanted to do was get through all of this, put the experience in a wooden box, bury it or sledgehammer it to bits when I had the strength. I heard that cancer is "the gift that keeps on giving." I hoped it would decide to be an "Indian giver" like the snot-nosed bully on the playground who bullies others with the "gift" of friendship. I was determined to make this a short-lived relationship and as soon as my ordeal was over, cancer could shove my friendship up its ass along with the splinters from the wooden box.

My oncologist decides to put me on a medication used for depression as it also acts as a nerve blocker. I hesitate to take it because one: I might be a little off my rocker but I'm not depressed, and two: one more pill to add to the spice rack of drugs may topple the whole thing over. And if my sleeping pills get lost at the bottle of the pile, I'm totally screwed because I can't sleep without one.

I take one of these pills in the morning, on a work day no less, and two hours later, I notice my pupils are dilated like I just revisited the sacred sorority bong. To add insult to injury, the image looking back at me in the mirror is that of a bald, stoned looking woman who can't walk. This is getting ridiculous. How much can a person take?

Wednesday, April 22, 2009 7:00 AM, CDT

The verdict is in on my Taxol treatments. As per my oncologist, "Too bad sister, you're still getting it." The leg pain has subsided, so that leads my doctor to believe that any further pain will not result in permanent damage to my legs. He said that my A-C treatments and the Taxol treatments are my best chance at a cure and he doesn't want to risk a reoccurrence by cutting back on the Taxol or changing the treatment regimen because of the leg pain. So, basically, I need to suck it up for the next few weeks.

In order to better deal with the leg pain, my doctor is going to prescribe Morphine to get me through. I said, "Great! Then I'll be like Gary Busey on *Celebrity Rehab* slurring and drooling all over myself." My doctor has assured me it will be a low dose to keep the pain at bay.

I can't believe that after tomorrow, I will be 75 percent DONE with my chemo. Every day has been a struggle, but it is going by and each day is getting me closer to the end. Thank goodness! My very last treatment is May 21st, and it will be here before I know it. My upcoming surgeries are going to feel like a tooth pull compared to the chemo I have been through.

I would not have been able to get this far had it not been for the love and support of Mark, my kids, my family and all of my friends.

I'll keep you posted on this next treatment.

Love, Connie

Wednesday, April 22, 2009 11:41 AM, CDT

Keep your chin up—you're almost there! I am thinking about you and looking forward to that cocktail. Have you gotten that massage yet???

Elena T.

Wednesday, April 22, 2009 11:50 AM, CDT

Dear Connie,

I am so sorry to hear about your leg pain. I'm praying for you and your family. You are mightily blessed with all the loving support of your family and friends. One day at a time...

Sending you a hug,

Love You, Maureen L.

Wednesday, April 22, 2009 1:23 PM, CDT

Miss Connie,

The photos are great!! Thanks for sharing. You are quite a woman to be going though all this and still have a sense of humor!!! Sometimes laughter is the best medicine. Sorry you have had to go through so much pain. I continue to think about you and pray for you and your family. Hang in there!!!

Debbie D.

Wednesday, April 22, 2009 2:29 PM, CDT

GO Connie Go Connie...OK that was me being a cheerleader...

Glad to see that you're doing better dealing with the leg pain...

I have to deal with a pain in my ass...(Jim) everyday :) so I kind of know what you're going thru LOL.

All kidding aside, you're in my prayers…

See you soon

Debra D.

Thursday, April 23, 2009 8:43 AM, CDT

Connie,

Glad to hear your leg pain has subsided…still keeping you in my thoughts and prayers!!!

Love,

Wendy C.

Thursday, April 23, 2009 1:58 PM, CDT

Connie,

Thinking of you!! xoxoxo Missy T.

I think at this point it would be helpful to have a Chemo Handbook. Not one written by a doctor in medical jargon, but one written by someone who experienced it and actually lived to tell about it. I'm all about contributing to the handbook, the best application of my literary skills to be used in the chapter entitled, "Feel Like Shit: Cocktails and Coping Strategies." I've got some great material. Somehow, I don't think the medical community would appreciate my tell-it-like-it-is approach.

Have I mentioned that morphine makes some people itch like rabid dogs with lice? Yeah, that would be me. It certainly helps with the pain but now when I wake up, I look like someone scrubbed my body in the night with that wire brush I never use to clean the grill. Maybe that damn thing is in my bedroom somewhere. I make a mental note to tie my hands together before I go to bed so I don't scratch the shit out of myself while I sleep.

Chapter 27
Laughter In The Commode

Thursday, April 23, 2009 11:20 AM, CDT

Today I went for chemo and when I met with my oncologist, he told me that he and the other doctors in the practice have discussed my severe leg-pain reaction to the Taxol and have decided to switch my chemo regimen. They are afraid that if they continue with the Taxol, I may have permanent nerve damage to my legs.

Good news, but also a major setback. Good news because I (hopefully) will not endure the horrific leg pain any longer, but bad news as this new treatment, Taxotere, will prolong my chemo. I still have 3 treatments left, but these need to be given once every three weeks (as opposed to every other). So they just added 10 more weeks to my treatment schedule. 10 MORE WEEKS!

What is so disappointing and depressing is that I had the end in sight. I was counting down the days. Keeping my eye on the prize. I was excited that my reconstructive surgery was just around the corner, I would have breasts for summer and would stop feeling so completely deformed and self-conscious. The day is coming, but the fact that it is now that much further out is such a mental blow.

I'm SO TIRED. Sick and tired of being sick and tired. I just want to crawl in a hole with a bowl of ice cream and escape all of this. I'm pissy and I've totally had it.

I know I will return to my positive-thinking self (maybe in a few days), but right now I am one upset, depressed and angry chick. Yes, I am grateful that I can beat this, but beating it is a mentally, physically and emotionally draining journey.

I will keep you all posted!

Love, Connie

Pissed is not anywhere near a word that could accurately describe where my head is at this point in time. When he was a kid, my brother had this Stretch Armstrong doll; you could (obviously) stretch out all of its limbs. I know I am dating myself here, but I feel like that doll with my arms, legs and head all stretched out and tied in a knot like a pretzel that leaves your mouth dry as a bone.

There is not one specific incident or experience in your life that can prepare you for this journey, just a compilation of events and situations stored neatly in a compartment that you can pull out of the card catalog when needed. And if you are a spaz like me, the cards are not so neatly arranged, more so like a six-year-old's version of the game 52 card pickup.

Oh to be six again. Even for just a day. Innocence rampant, maturity elusive for many years, and depending on the person, possibly decades away. About a year before I was diagnosed, my marital separation was new and like the first days of rainy crappy spring. My daughter was at a Girl Scout shindig and I asked Alex what he wanted to do and he said, "Let's go to Friendly's." Little did I know that this was a restaurant visit we would talk about for YEARS.

We arrived, grabbed a booth, and immediately, Alex had to go to the bathroom. OF COURSE he had to go to the bathroom! I thought that maybe when he turned 8, he'd decide that "testing out" the bathroom of EVERY destination was getting a little old. We took said trip to the ladies room. As we walked in, this elderly woman stepped in and I motioned for her to go in front of me and use the handicap stall, while Alex was in the other stall. So immediately upon dropping trow, this poor woman launched into a cacophony of flatulence that was just, well, astounding. I thought, "Oh, please God, Alex don't say anything. Don't laugh. Just be quiet and pee!" As I tried to restrain my laughter, I said to Alex, "Hey Bud, how are you doing?"

"Gooooood," he said. I knew the kid was just about to have a breakdown because the woman was tooting up a storm. If we could have added a snare drum and a bass guitar, we could have easily had a three piece band and maybe a #1 song, "The Fart Song."

A woman walked in with her three little girls, stood for a moment, heard the music and raised an eyebrow at me. Her daughter said, "Mommy, what is THAT noise?" She quickly ushered them out and I was left with my six-year-old son behind a closed door praying he would not laugh. Finally, he opened the door with this shit-eating grin and I put my finger to my mouth and quietly said, "Don't you laugh!" He laughed as he washed his hands and I held my hand over his mouth to stop the noise while his little shoulders moved up and down with his laughter. Oh, to have been a fly on the wall. We couldn't make it two minutes through our lunch without bursting into laughter!

I realize that life will throw me curve balls like cancer. But it's the little moments like the farting old lady that get you through. If you are lucky, there are many little moments that make you smile and appreciate your journey. I am so hoping that Alex always remembers the farting old lady and that my illness, and all that goes with it, is a fading memory.

Chapter 28

The Home Stretch

Thursday, April 30, 2009 4:47 PM, CDT

I survived treatment #6 today! I am 75 percent of the way there! The doctor I saw today told me that if I have the same type of reaction to this chemo, he would recommend that I discontinue with my chemo. But he is not my doctor, so we'll have to see. I have a wonderful doctor, but he's more along the lines of a "suck it up and deal with it" doctor, so I'm thinking I've got 2 more rounds of this fun stuff.

My two favorite nurses came over to administer my poison and I said, "Here come the sisters of death." They laughed. We always have a good laugh while I am there. It is the only thing that helps to keep me sane when they start poking me with needles!

I feel fine right now, just a bit tired and very hot from all of the steroids I have to take for this chemo. Maybe I should try to pull together enough energy to work out and build some muscle mass. Need to take advantage of the 'roids!

I am having the hot flashes associated with menopause (fun), but they tell me it is a "false menopause" until my chemo is over…OR NOT. It could be permanent. I remember when my Mom had hot flashes and we would laugh about it because she would act like a crazy person fanning herself. Well, they are not fun, so I'm hoping it goes away SOON! I'm already crazy enough.

I'm so glad the weather is getting better. I have been trying to get out and walk when I feel well enough. It has been very hard for me to be sedentary for so long. I'm jumping out of my skin. If this chemo works, there are 3 weeks in between it and the next round, so I hope that will give me one solid week in the middle where I feel great and can get out and do things. The kids have been so understanding of my circumstances. We are working on plans to do things when I am better, so we are excited about that.

I should know by Saturday if I am in the clear with the leg pain, as last time it happened two days after chemo. Tomorrow I have to go back and have the Neulasta shot to help with my bone marrow production and white blood cell count. I am not looking forward to it, as it makes my body ache for DAYS!

I hope you are all doing well and enjoying the nice weather. FINALLY! I will keep you posted!

Love, Connie :)

Friday, April 24, 2009 6:03 AM, CDT

Connie,

I'm sorry to hear of your setback. I'm sure it would piss me off as well. You have every right to feel that way. This will be done soon. You'll be on a beach somewhere looking hot in your bikini, :) feeling great and playing with your kids. Keep your faith and your sense of humor!

If I can do anything for you, please let me know.

Love,

Bev B.

Friday, April 24, 2009 11:59 AM, CDT

Hey Connie,

So sorry to hear about this latest setback…but I am sure it will only make you stronger. Believe it or not, I think about you often and send only good wishes your way.

Lauren J.

Friday, April 24, 2009 10:01 PM, EDT

I wanna kick cancer' s ass!!!!!

Kurt B.

Sunday, April 26, 2009 9:14 PM, CDT

Oh CRAP!! You deserve 2 be pissed off and tired. Please tell me you are cutting yourself some slack and trying to rest. I know you want to keep a "stiff upper lip" for everyone and keep going like the energizer bunny you are, but know when you need to take a break, too, OK? I have you in my thoughts every day. Love, Jen K.

Tuesday, April 28, 2009 7:46 PM, CDT

Hey Connie,

I am so sorry that I have not been around. I think of you all of the time and you are in my prayers and thoughts. It is OK to be pissed off. You will kick this in the butt...I still plan on drinking a beer with you in October.

Love,

SueAnn L.

Thursday, April 30, 2009 7:47 PM, CDT

Hey Connie. I know that you are so used to being the one with the "get up and go" but rest is just as important. Think about a warm place to go when this is all over. You and the kids deserve a vacation! Think of you often and you remain in my prayers. Love In/Out Judy G.

Thursday, April 30, 2009 8:08 PM, CDT

Hey Connie—

You are in my thoughts and prayers every day and I have been following your progress. I hope you make it up to P'burgh in October—should be lots of fun this year. Keep up your great attitude and take care of yourself.

Margaret C.

Thursday, April 30, 2009 9:05 PM, CDT

Hey Connie,

I'm glad today went OK. I will be praying for you that you don't have the leg pain and that you can get on with your last 2 treatments and be done with this!

Take care and I'll talk to you soon,

Love,

Mary Beth F.

Friday, May 1, 2009 6:20 AM, CDT

Connie,

I hope this new chemo works for you. With all the needles, it sounds like you could be a pincushion!! There is light at the end of the tunnel!! Every day that goes by is one day closer to being finished with all your treatments. I'm so glad that your children are doing well with all you've been through and that you all have a bright future ahead where you can get out and enjoy life.

All the best to you.

Debbie D.

Friday, May 1, 2009 1:51 PM, CDT

Connie,

Just wanted to let you know I am thinking about you!!

Keep your eyes on the prize. Take a deep breath and enjoy the day. If I haven't told you lately...you are such an incredible blessing to all of us on this site.

Love ya.

Lisa D.

Saturday, May 2, 2009 10:56 AM, CDT

Hey there lady,

I think about you often. I wish I could see you more. Hang in there and get through this. We are all pulling for you. Hope to see you soon.

Love Ya!

Kellie H.

Chapter 29
Menopause and Other Fun Stuff

*T*he word "menopause" is not typically a conversation starter, nor is "I have my period." But it all starts somewhere in our younger years, maybe fifth grade, when we girls receive "the talk" from the school nurse while the boys are ushered out to the playground for extra recess.

Michelle was my best friend growing up and her mom was the school nurse. My mother was the substitute school nurse.

The day arrived for the much-anticipated talk and Michelle looked at me and said, "I don't think my mother is here today."

"WHAAAT?" I said. My mind was completely frantic! Holy shit, is MY mother giving the talk? We heard the cart rolling down the hallway, I looked at Michelle and held my breath.

"Hello girls!" Sure as shit, it was my mother, there to give the dreaded talk of the period to the entire class. My mother was a very private person. We never really talked about this stuff and we especially didn't talk about sex. So I pretty much died when she asked, "Does anyone use tampons?"

I would later find out that my mother had something of an obsession with tampons. Like there was going to a world drought of cotton with a string attached. She would visit me at college and bring me ten boxes at a time. I would say, "Mom, I'm going to be home in three months! I think three boxes are fine." And she would say, "Well you always want to be prepared." Yeah, maybe if my hot water heater blew, I could sop up all of the water with tampons.

Let me put it this way—in my early twenties, my boyfriend opened my closet door and said, "Jesus, are you supplying tampons for everyone in New York State?"

To hear of my impending menopause and "change of life" is a bit startling. Hot flashes, bitchiness (more so than usual), no more tampons, how is a girl to cope? Don't old ladies go through this? I know my kids think I'm old, but what do they know? When my oncologist initially went over my treatment plan, five years of hormone therapy was part of my cure cocktail. I was vehemently opposed to this from the beginning, as the cure it helped to foster brought along with it side effects that have proven deadly. My mother had taken Tamoxifen and had died from what we thought was a uterine mass, so to repeat history even further than it was already written, wasn't part of the story I had intended to write for myself. I was determined that my story would have a different ending.

Ultimately, my treatment plan is MY decision. I know that I infuriated my oncologist with my "I'm not doing this and I'm not doing that" mentality. If I didn't have that one damn microscopic bit of cancer in my lymph node, we wouldn't even be discussing hormone therapy. I'd have a new rack, still have my hair and we'd have called it a day. Put a big 'ol period at the end of the cancer story.

Well, as always, wishful thinking.

Monday, May 4, 2009 10:14 PM, CDT

I have a strong dislike for tequila. It couldn't possibly have anything to do with the worm mishap, where one slid down my throat in college on a dare, followed by a lot of yakking. Having said that, Jose Cuervo and I may need to become fast friends again because the leg pain is back with a vengeance and there doesn't seem to be an appropriate narcotic in my spice rack of meds. It's like a million chemo Nazis poking holes in my legs with daggers, making my legs like Swiss cheese. I like cheese, but not Swiss!

When I asked my doctor last week what the difference was between Taxol (the first leg pain chemo) and Taxotere (the NEW leg pain chemo), he said, "Well, the Taxotere attacks the cancer at the microtubule level, blah, blah, blah."

I looked at him pan-faced and said, "I don't give a shit about microtubules! How's it going to make me FEEL?" Apparently, THE SAME!

The only difference is that I had a couple of good days in between. Which is a total plus, because I got a lot done around the house and Mark and I took the kids to the carnival in Clifton Park on Saturday and we had a great time. There were no wig/ride mishaps to be caught on *America's Funniest Home Videos.* Having a wig gets you out of having to go on "Zero Gravity" with your kids. BONUS!

I bought some hanging flowers for my porch over the weekend and they are beautiful. I was looking out one of my front windows at the flowers today thinking, "I am so grateful to be here looking at these flowers." But I have to admit that I feel like the chick from the indoor/outdoor allergy commercial, where she has one foot on each side. I have one foot on "Grateful to be here, am going to survive" and the other foot on "Are you kidding me? Make it stop! Make it stop!" Is there an end in sight? Am I ever going to wake up and not think about being a cancer patient first thing in the morning when my feet hit the floor? Yes and yes, but it isn't going to happen as fast as an allergy pill, that's for sure. This whole experience is definitely (trying to) teach me patience.

I'm sick of being the bald chick I catch in the mirror (in the privacy of my own home of course). The girl I affectionately refer to as Uncle Fester's sister. Uncle Fester's sister, who is of course, BALD, but ironically enough has to use a Schick razor to shave her legs! Wasn't the one small bonus of chemo supposed to be NOT HAVING TO SHAVE YOUR LEGS?

Speaking of hairy, Mark bought the kids hamsters today. They are thrilled! The kids, I mean. The hamsters, I don't know. All I could think about today was my own childhood hamster mishap (I have a lot of mishaps) where my hamster got loose, ran into the heating duct and died there in the middle of winter. The smell could have killed a pack of rabid wolves. If my mother were alive, she'd say, "We're making memories!"

We are making memories! I just hope that the kids remember all of the funny things we have done during my illness and not the illness. Doesn't cancer realize I am a mom who has stuff to do? I have kickball games to lose, not LOSE because I can't run the bases! The hardest part of all is not knowing day-to-day how I am going to feel. It's definitely hard for "the planner" to plan anything. The kids have been troopers through this whole thing and on this Mother's Day, I am truly grateful for smart, loving kids, who love their mom no matter what she's dealing with. As Alex often says, "Mom, you're the best Mom ever...even when you yell." Now that's a kid who loves me! LOL.

I hope all of my amazing friends who are moms have a wonderful Mother's Day!

Much love to all, Connie :)

Tuesday, May 5, 2009 6:30 AM, CDT

Connie, I was so hoping that this chemo treatment would be better for you. Hopefully the side effect doesn't last as long. You are almost there. It will be over soon. You are so strong. I don't think I could look at this situation the way you do. You see humor and you laugh. You see so much in life and your family and they are helping you through this. I feel God gave you these kids with such big hearts for a reason. They give you pieces of their hearts everyday to strengthen yours. Take each day one hour at a time. And please do not go swallowing any worms…remember you do not like the vomiting effect of choking on it. Think of you very often. Love Judy G.

Tuesday, May 5, 2009 8:03 AM, CDT

Connie,

I'm telling you, if you published these journals into a book I could see you sitting on the couch of *The Today Show* being interviewed by Matt Lauer a year from now. You are a fantastic writer. Sorry to hear about the leg pain. Call me later. I'm up for drinks next Wednesday. It's on the calendar!!!! Hamsters???? Jason will take the hermit crabs if it gets to be too much work.

Rene S.

Tuesday, May 5, 2009 9:13 AM, CDT

> Con—
>
> I love you more than words can say!!!!
>
> I am sorry to hear that the second course was as painful as the first especially after waiting so long in-between!!
>
> You are blessed with a multitude of good things and people around you!!! Have a WONDERFUL MOTHER'S DAY !!!
>
> Always thinking of you— LOL—Michelle H.

Mother's Day comes and I think of my mother. I contemplate going to the cemetery to visit her grave, to talk to her in some way, knowing that each time I go, I am ruined for days. Her death is so real when I read her name on the stone. I cry for days and I think, "Would she want me to be like this?"

Years before, the kids maybe three and four, Derek and I went to her grave to place flowers. He walked the kids back to the car while I sat at her gravesite quietly telling her how much I missed her, how beautiful her grandchildren were. I sat there and cried, completely inconsolable. I felt drained as if she had died all over again. I can say with complete clarity that my mother's death is something I will never get over. It will stay with me forever, but I know that it makes me stronger.

Kids are awesome. So completely uncensored. The day after visiting my mother's grave, Alyssa was sitting on my bed reading a *Winnie the Pooh* book, talking to me as she perused the pages and I stood in my bathroom putting on mascara. "Mom, Grandma Jackie was sick right?"

"Yes honey."

"And then she died."

"That's right."

"And then she dug a big hole and got into a scasket (casket)."

"Kind of." Oh my God, where is she getting this from?

"Well, I'll tell you Mom, she's not getting out of that hole!"

Oh My God! I had to go hide in my closet and laugh in private. If my mother were alive, she would have totally laughed her ass off! I called my dad to tell him and he was completely mortified. My brother, however, saw the humor and immediately said, "Mom would have really gotten a kick out of that."

A few days later, I was making the kids lunch and Alyssa asked me, "Mom, does Grandma Jackie eat lunch down in the hole?"

"No honey, Grandma Jackie doesn't each lunch anymore."

Life is so terribly fragile. And yet, while we're here, we meet people who have insurmountable strength: strength of character, physical will to live and belief in the love of others. People who bless you with their very existence and whose absence in death leaves a void that nothing can fill. My mother was this person to me, and to so many others. Yes, life is fragile, short and unfair. And there are definitely no more peanut butter and jelly sandwiches to be shared.

I am so close to the end of this journey. Well, at least I'm hopeful that the end is nearing. I'm not going to lie, I have wrestled with my own mortality. It's inevitable with any cancer diagnosis I think. Like peering down the barrel of a shotgun, half expecting it to go off. I'd like to think I have taken on cancer and kicked its ass.

For me, and for my mother.

Chapter 30
Kiss Off, Chemo!

Wednesday, May 6, 2009 2:43 PM, CDT

I AM DONE WITH CHEMO!! I AM DONE WITH CHEMO!! I just got back from the oncologist and he said that my leg pain reaction is a level of toxicity to chemo that he has never seen and he does not want to continue for fear of permanent damage to my legs.

I AM SO HAPPY! I have been feeling like this was never going to be over. Now I just have some surgeries and hormone therapy ahead.

My doctor gave me morphine for the leg pain. I think I might have a drink to celebrate (and maybe a morphine too)!

Love to all!! Con :)

Wednesday, May 6, 2009 3:03 PM, CDT

Yay! Congratulations! Mixing the morphine and a cocktail sounds like fun. I want you up in Saratoga for that massage (*she was so sweet to buy me a gift certificate*) and a cocktail! Please let me know when you think you can do it. In the mean time, have a wonderful rest of your week and a wonderful Mother's Day. Looking forward to seeing you.

Elena T.

Wednesday, May 6, 2009 3:44 PM, CDT

Hurray...whoop de doo...great gads a-fire...wonderful wonderful and celebration is needed...have a drink or two, eat hearty, if you are feeling like it, go out for dinner. Have yourself a good ole' time. I am so happy for you: this is a wonderful day...for all of us who love you too. Now, on to getting the boobs back...I hope you looked at the catalog information I sent to you on your personal e-mail.

Take care and give big hugs to the kids.

Dotte C.

Wednesday, May 6, 2009 4:10 PM, CDT

Connie,

Woo Hoo!!! Yes, there is light at the end of the tunnel!!! Way to go... looking back at all that you have endured, you are a remarkable woman!!! Have a blessed Mother's Day.

Debbie D.

Wednesday, May 6, 2009 4:34 PM, CDT

Thank God! So sorry this one was again so tough...so glad you are done with this phase and can get on with things. We'll have to get together and celebrate!!

If I don't talk with you before, Happy Mother's Day. Talk to you soon!

Love,

Mary Beth F.

Wednesday, May 6, 2009 5:48 PM, CDT

Connie,

So thrilled to hear about the end of chemo. May you have a wonderful Mother's Day. Your mom would be so proud of you. You have gone through this with grace and humor. Feel good and I hope to talk to you soon!

Love,

SueAnn L.

Wednesday, May 6, 2009 5:59 PM, CDT

Ya Freakin Hoooo!!!!

Deana L.

Wednesday, May 6, 2009 9:27 PM, CDT

Connie,

So happy to hear this great news!! Now we can start planning that visit! Miss you and know that you will continue to get stronger every day!

xoxo, Britt B.

Thursday, May 7, 2009 4:50 AM, CDT

WOOOOOHOOOOO!!!!!!!!!!!!!!!!!!!!!!!!!!! I'm dancing… what awesome news, Con!!! You have got to be ready to just jump out of your skin with joy! OK, onward we go!!!

What a great Mother's Day gift to you; I love you so much and hope you have the most memorable Mother's Day.

My prayers, positive thoughts and hugs keep coming your way— from my heart to yours.

XOXOXOXOXO

Kathy S.

Thursday, May 7, 2009 5:45 AM, CDT

WOOT WOOT!!!! What fantastic news! I'm so happy you're done and can move on. I hope your leg pain sub-sides soon and you feel fantastic :) Have a wonderful Mother's Day.

You remain an inspiration to all!

Love,

Bev B.

Thursday, May 7, 2009 9:05 AM, CDT

I have been waiting to hear those very words! That is fan-tastic news. Some surgery and a few visits w/ Dr. Mark (*therapist*) and you'll be better than ever. Now it's really time for a visit. I'll still clean your toilet with your tub brush when I visit…can't break a tradition.

Joan F.

Thursday, May 7, 2009 8:10 PM, CDT

Thank Goodness it is finally behind you!!!!!!!!! I am so proud of you. You got through it. May your journey now be an easy and less-painful one. Still thinking of you. Judy G.

Friday, May 8, 2009 12:07 PM, CDT

YEAAAAAAA!!!!! How great to hear!!!!! Celebrate with your all, Connie! Only good news ahead! Love, Anna B.

Friday, May 8, 2009 3:58 PM, CDT

Woo hoo!!!!! I am so happy for you!!! I guess something good comes out of something bad again...I had a salamander when I was a kid that crawled in the heating vent and roasted and that too left an odor in the house for weeks that I will never forget ...funny!

I am happy you are here too and hope your summer is a great one...miss you

Jen K.

Sunday, May 10, 2009 7:51 AM, EDT

HAPPY MOTHER'S DAY, my dear friend!!! Cherish each moment today and hold it close to your heart. You are a phenomenal woman, who is an inspiration to all. Your children are such a tribute to who you are.

I hope your day will be filled with laughter and sunshine. I love you. Prayers, hugs and positive energy from my heart to yours,

Kathy S.

I leave the oncologist's office with an incredible sense of self-satisfaction, as if I was giving cancer the middle finger. I can compare the feeling to the fantasy every woman has of running into an ex. Imagine the scene.

You walk into a crowded bar wearing an amazing red dress, your hair perfectly coiffed. You see him standing at the bar amid a handful of friends. He acknowledges you, so you walk over. He says, "Wow, you look AMAZING!" You fumble in your purse saying, "I thought I had a lollipop in here for you because you still SUCK, right? You turn on your heel and walk away to the sound of laughter from his friends and smile at the thought of his facing turning as red as your dress. OK, so that's MY fantasy. We're all entitled to one, right?

To celebrate the end of chemo, I decide to get a spray tan. I've never had one, and as I pull into the tanning salon, I have visions of walking out jaundiced, looking like an oompa loompa. Most of my girlfriends have gotten them and I chuckle as I remember a summer event a couple of years ago where one of my friends had her spray tan dripping off her from the heat. It's only May, so no need to fear the melt.

I haven't been to the tanning salon in quite a while, so when I walk in with my wig on, they know no different. The girl tells me to make sure I wear the shower cap, rub the lotion provided on my fingers and toes so as to avoid the orange jaundice in my cuticle beds and press the button when I'm ready to rock. I take my wig off, throw the shower cap on and head in for my spray tan. I get out, rub the excess off and just about DIE when I look in the mirror. What the FUCK was I thinking wearing a shower cap on a BALD HEAD?? A perfectly tanned, nipple-less body is looking back at me with a completely white bald head that could corral cattle into a stable like a beacon!

I get home and as I look in my bathroom mirror, I can hear my mother's uproarious laugh, only to realize that it is ME laughing at myself. My neighbor Kim is driving by and waves to me while I'm outside. She stops and I tell her that she HAS to come in and see something. We sit in my dining room, and as I take my wig off to show her the aftermath of my tanning adventure, we laugh so hard we can barely breathe. My daughter comes in. Kim and I are cracking up as I struggle to get my wig back on my head. Alyssa stands there with her mouth agape, and I know if she were permitted, she would have said, "WTF?" Instead, she looks at me and says, "Mom, you're nuts!" Yeah, I know. I KNOW!

I made an attempt to be a stay-at-home mom when the kids were two and three years old. It was exhausting and I probably cried every day. Hats off to stay-at-home moms because it is hard work! Anyway, I was cooking dinner one afternoon, alone with the kids, and Abe got out of the house. His escapes were similar to a greyhound's reaction to the opening of a gate, followed by a cat-and-mouse scenario to catch him that usually ended with my walking away to have a glass of wine. Without Abe.

He decides to have a standoff with Kim's dog on her front lawn, and proceeds to dig himself into her mulch. As I approach him, he flicks a TON of mulch on her porch with his feet as he runs away. After dinner that night, I grab a broom and tell the kids we're taking a walk. We walk over to Kim's house, and as the kids sit on her lawn, I proceed to sweep her porch free of mulch. Just as I am mid-sweep, her husband, who DOES NOT KNOW ME, drives up to the house with a "WTF is going on here" look. I explain myself, finish sweeping and as we're heading home Alyssa says, "Mom, whose porch are we sweeping next?"

As we sat there laughing at my white head, the realization hit that I'd be back to sweeping porches in no time. Happy, healthy and sweeping mulch off of porches!

Chapter 31
A ThreeFer

Thursday, May 14, 2009 2:50 PM, CDT

Lots of news to share…First, Mark bought me a puppy. A Lhasa Apso (or so we were told), cute as all-get-out. We named him "Chemo" because we wanted to replace the real chemo with something happy. Something happy that pees and poops every 5 seconds and finds the craziest places that are unreachable to make his "deposits." It's like *War of the Roses* in my house between a 3 lb. dog and Abe, our 90 lb. chocolate lab. Abe's face is so expressive, you can't help but KNOW what he's thinking. He looks at Chemo like, "Are you kidding me? You're staying?" With the two dogs, along with the two hamsters, two hermit crabs and two kids, I've got my own version of Noah's Ark.

I went to my oncologist yesterday and I don't have to go back for 3 months!! 3 months!! We talked about my starting on Tamoxifen (the hormone therapy—I worked him for 2 weeks off so I start June 1st) and we discussed my thyroid situation. I asked him for my thyroid ultrasound film so I could take it to my surgeon and he looked in my chart and said, "Looks like they sent it to my brother's office." So his brother is a doctor of infectious medicine.

I said, "Your parents must be very proud." He said yes and I said, "They must REALLY brag about YOU. 'My son Ed poisons people and makes them cry.'" We had a good laugh over that. It has to be difficult being an oncologist and he is such a great doctor—I really have had fantastic care.

Today I saw the surgeon who specializes in thyroid surgery. He examined me and recommended doing a needle biopsy on a large nodule I have on my left side. I said, "Then what?" He told me it would probably need to be taken out whether it is cancer or not because it is so large. So I said, "What are we messing around with a needle biopsy for then?" The breast biopsy was like poking your eye with a needle and having it come out your nose, so why would I want to have a long needle stuck in my neck? Just the thought of it makes me want to pass out. So the long and the short of it is that on June 3rd I am having half my thyroid removed (the other half as well if the nodule is cancerous), my chemo port removed and my chest expander put back in my right side. I told the surgeon, "This is like one-stop shopping at Wal-Mart. Buy a garden hose, buy a frozen pizza; get a boob back, take out a thyroid. Same kind of deal."

He said the thyroid surgery will affect my voice, making it hoarser (maybe I'll sound sexier) and I won't be able to yell for awhile. I said, "I know a 7 year old and an 8 year old who'll be very happy about that!" I'll have to make signs that say "GO TO YOUR ROOM," "BECAUSE I SAID SO," "GET YOUR PAJAMAS ON—NOW," "DINNER'S READY" and on and on. It'll be my own version of "flashcards." It'll be interesting, that's for sure.

I am one happy chick. I am almost done with this journey to wellness. Still a bit tired and coming out of my chemo fog, but definitely on the mend. I'm so thankful to be here, honestly. And mostly thankful for all of my amazing friends, my family and especially Mark for sticking by me through all of this mess.

I hope this note finds you all well. I'm going to make myself a pomegranate martini and call it a day. After all, it's 5 o'clock SOMEWHERE.

Love, Connie :)

Thursday, May 14, 2009 5:10 PM, CDT

Yeah, Connie! You sound so great and still with such a sense of humor that I am laughing out loud as I read through your letter!

After all you have been through the rest will be a breeze... and will be over in no time! I understand the needles and when you think in visuals...it is a bit much! Love, Anna B.

Thursday, May 14, 2009 7:23 PM, CDT

Loving this update! Thanks for sharing and making us laugh!

Joan F.

Thursday, May 14, 2009 10:50 PM, CDT

Great news! So glad to hear you are at the end of all of this.

Your spirit and sense of humor throughout this continues to be amazing.

Have fun with Chemo!

Mary Beth F.

Friday, May 15, 2009 8:43 AM, CDT

Connie,

You never cease to amaze me!! It was so nice to hear all your good news and you have such a wonderful sense of humor!!

I too have a problem with my thyroid. I have goiters on mine. I have been taking Tamoxifen for almost a year now.

Keep up your good spirits and I look forward to hearing more great news.

Have a blessed day!!

Debbie D.

Friday, May 15, 2009 10:09 AM, CDT

You go girl...you take it all in stride and deal with what is at hand each day. I had almost forgotten the thyroid thing. It is good to get that out of the way...then you can be on to a fabulous spring. I am so happy for you that things have progressed so well.

Keep up the humor...I'm sure the doctors are amused by you...and probably tell the other doctors about you.

We will all be anxious until we hear the results of the thyroid and pray it is nothing to worry about.

Dotte C.

Saturday, May 16, 2009 5:44 PM, CDT

Con— I had sooo much fun the other day !! We definitely need to do that again!!!! I am sooo HAPPY to hear that you don't need to go back for another three months!!! Please don't concentrate on the thyroid thing!! If you need to be on synthroid for the rest of your life, I can tell you first-hand, it's nothing!! I love ya lots and I hope to see you soon!!

Michelle H.

Sunday, May 17, 2009 7:48 AM, EDT

Oh, Con…how you make me laugh!!!! What amazingly GREAT NEWS!! If I know you, you'll have Chemo trained to seek, find and clean up his own deposits before long. With all of the challenges you have met and conquered in the past 7 months, house-training Chemo will be a breeze.

You sound soooo awesome and this wonderful news has got to put a little extra ooomph into your never-ending spirit. You'll have to take some pictures of Chemo and Abe and post them.

Keep your mind on the prize my dear friend, you are almost there. I love you; positive thoughts, prayers and hugs from my heart to yours… XOXOXO Kathy S.

The days leading up to this next surgery are filled with a mixture of excitement and dread. Excitement at the thought of getting on with things; my next step in the journey. Dread knowing that the beginning of many surgeries is about to commence.

As I came out of what my oncologist coined "the chemo fog," I began to see many of my struggles with a great deal of clarity. Had I been through hell?

ABSOFREAKINLUTELY! Was I OK? YES. Did I have more to come? Well, DUH! But, I was through the worst of it, physically that is. Emotionally, I faced so much more.

My relationship with Mark is in a bad place. His disappearances are more frequent, his presence more absent. I put on a smile, but I know where things are headed. My good health is just around the corner, and I am hoping for so much more. The sun will come out and before me will be a beautiful rainbow, along with the ever-expected pot of gold, with many good times ahead. During my chemo, I had imagined myself feeling better; Mark and I back to the fun relationship we once had.

I am intuitive. I AM a woman. It's my job to be, isn't it? Eh, I'll just deal with it all later. I push the negative into a little compartment in my mind that I try to bury until I get through the next onslaught of "happy juice" and scalpels. It will be there later, for sure.

The thought of being whole again is within reach. I am excited at the thought of ending my one-titted wonderness. The days of stuffing one side of my chest everyday with gauze are coming to an end. It's funny to me to think that I was so self-conscious about this. Always careful to hug people so they wouldn't feel the flatness of my chest.

The chemo port protrusion from my chest is to be replaced with a more normal protrusion. Now I can wear a tank-top, or a bathing suit and no one is going to ask, "What the hell is that hexagon shaped thing in your chest?" As I prepare for my next surgery, I feel a sense of relief that I am one step closer to not being sick anymore.

Sunday, June 7, 2009 6:06 PM, CDT

Wow! It's been awhile since I've written in my journal! I had my 3-in-1 surgery last Wednesday and I'm SO GLAD it's over. I won't know the exact pathology of my thyroid for a week or so, but the surgeon told me he is 95 percent sure it is not cancer. So that's good news. I had my chemo port taken out and my breast expander put back in on my right side (I have my boobs back!).

The outcome was not quite what I had expected. My throat looks like I have been in a slasher movie and I happened to be at the wrong place at the wrong time when Freddy Krueger was in town. I look like one of those apples I try to convince my kids are OK to eat because they have all of the bad spots cut away. Just another of many battle scars to show that I have endured this journey.

I am very sore. I seem to have also had a run-in with a Mack truck while I was under the knife. This too, shall pass. Nothing a couple of good narcotics can't fix!

The surgeon had told me prior to my surgery that my voice may be affected. I told him that I was going to come out of this surgery the perfect girlfriend for Mark. I was getting a new boob (so I would have two, BONUS!) and would have no voice. LOL! We had a good laugh over that. Fortunately, my voice was not affected so I didn't have to make up a bunch of flash cards for the kids saying, "Because I said so" or "Go to bed NOW." Honestly, I would have been too tired to even make them up. I would have had to resort to hand gestures. And that would have been a dangerous combination with the narcotics I'm on. All's well that ends well there.

The only issue I had in the hospital was that my blood pressure was extremely low (for me). It was 80/54, so they were on a mission to pump me full of fluids to get it back up to an acceptable level. Let me put it to you this way: I had so much fluid in me, I felt like a raft inflated with air, certain that I would have had enough buoyancy to float down the Hudson River, through the locks to Manhattan and get back home WITHOUT a life preserver. I have to be the only chick on the planet who can go into the hospital and come out 24 hours later weighing 10 lbs more! Good grief!

I haven't totally lost my wits. They asked me as they were rolling me back to my room what I wanted to drink and I asked for a Cosmopolitan. Beats hospital ginger ale, that's for sure.

As my mother would say, "Con Bramer, you're on the mend!" I am on the mend and all of this complete CRAZINESS that has CONSUMED my life and the lives of my loved ones will soon be over. One more surgery to get my implants and then have my nipples tattooed on (I still cannot believe this), and I AM DONE!

I look back on all of this and I realize that in the grand scheme of things, it has only been seven months since my diagnosis. Seven months is like a blip on your calendar of life. Big deal.

When you're a kid, time seems to take FOREVER. You can't wait to be in the double digits, you can't wait to graduate from high school, then college. And all of the sudden, quicker than you can even imagine, time flies by and you think "Holy crap, seven MONTHS just went by." The ONLY thing that I have experienced in my life to make time slow is facing a disease and having to live with it every day. Every moment. From the blink of your eyes to the morning sun to your last blink in the darkness before falling asleep.

Therein lies the challenge. To live with it, but not LIVE with it. My relationship with cancer is coming to an end. Like any relationship that is one-sided, there has to be an end. The difference being that I had to fight this "relationship" for seven months. It has been exhausting. Physically, mentally and emotionally. A fight worth fighting just the same. And all I can think about as my relationship with cancer ends, is all of the people who, unlike me, have an ongoing relationship with an antagonist that literally gnaws at them morning, noon and night. These are the people I think about and pray for every day.

I have been beyond blessed. Blessed with a great support system. Great friends, wonderful children, an amazing man to stand by my side and a family that would have done anything they could to take all of this away. I am so grateful. Thank you all for your messages, cards, thoughts and prayers and especially the laughter, because that's what has kept me going.

Thank you all so much for sharing my journey with me. I can't imagine going through this without all of you. As always, I will keep you posted.

Love, Connie :)

Sunday, June 7, 2009 7:15 PM, CDT

Congrats on a successful surgery! I am looking forward to my Cosmopolitan—with you, in Saratoga! Let me know when you're up to it!

Thinking about you,

Elena T.

Sunday, June 7, 2009 7:33 PM, CDT

Hey Connie,

So glad to hear you are on the mend from your surgeries and have another step behind you. I will look forward to seeing you soon and celebrating. Rest up and feel better.

You are amazing—you continue to handle all this with such strength, wisdom and humor. I am proud of you!!

Take care-

Love,

Mary Beth F

Monday, June 8, 2009 9:24 AM, CDT

Hey girlie. You are in the homestretch now!! Glad to hear you haven't lost your wits as you call them. That's why I fell in love with you after all. Let me know when you are ready for an outing or a visit. I am all moved in to my new house and am sending address change info to everyone today. Would love to have you over soon. Keep up those spirits!! Love you, Jen K.

Monday, June 8, 2009 4:13 PM, CDT

What a great message to read! I can't believe it's been 7 months! I feel like it was yesterday when we spoke and I said "In seven months most of this will be behind you." I am so proud of you and your courage has been mind-blowing. Can't wait to celebrate alongside you!

Joan F.

Monday, June 8, 2009 8:35 PM, CDT

Oh Connie, I am so happy for you. 7 months of ups and downs and even sideways if possible, and it is finally going to be behind you.

You need to know how inspirational you have been to all of us who at times thought our little things were major while you were fighting with all you had. Allowing us in and letting us know how your journey was going made me proud to call you my sister and my friend. You did it with such grace and laughter, even when doing so was rough.

Here is to that cosmopolitan that you so deserve. I wish I could come have one with you right now, but it will need to wait till October. I look forward to celebrating with you.

Heal from all of this and give those wonderful children one big hug.

Love In/Out Judy G.

Tuesday, June 9, 2009 1:42 PM, CDT

Connie

Another milestone…I have missed your messages and I just e-mailed you to see how the thyroid test came out. I hope it is benign…I thought maybe you had given up the Caring Bridge since we had not had a message for awhile.

I am so happy you got a boob and I'm sure your hair is growing back…at least I hope so.

Your sense of humor is so encouraging to all of us. I can't believe you have been through 7 months of this nasty stuff…but you are strong and beautiful…love Dotte C.

Another surgery down. A "three-fer." It is so great to have a chest again, and an even bigger bonus to be rid of the ever-annoying port. On the flip side, I have a horrendous gash in my neck from the thyroid surgery. A gash so ugly that a woman in Target ushered her daughter from me so quickly in line, she must have thought it was self-inflicted. Hey lady, yeah, I tried to slit my own throat! What is wrong with people?

Having this surgery behind me is freeing. Like an actual recovery is in sight. The journey has seemed so slow, and I am hopeful that the day-to-day grind of doctor visits and worry is edging closer to an end.

I finally feel like the puzzle pieces are coming together. For my health anyway. My relationship has pieces that just don't fit, and the more I try to push them together, the more frayed the edges become.

Chapter 32
Pain and Healing

Sunday, June 14, 2009 1:45 PM, CDT

Healing. What a loaded word. You fall down, you break your arm and it heals. Your doctor says, "Your cast can come off in 6 weeks." It has a timeline. The cast comes off, you figure you're HEALED.

Healing from cancer is a long, slow process. The physical scars may eventually fade to a tiny thin line, but the experience is like a cut that scabs over and over and over. And you start to wonder: is this the last scab?

Just like my relationship with cancer is coming to an end, so is my relationship with my boyfriend. I am grateful to him in so many ways for sticking by my side through so much. I know it had to be difficult to care about someone through a nasty divorce and then immediately following, cancer. It has been too much for me to bear at times, I can't imagine how difficult it has been for him.

I know it hasn't been easy for awhile. I have felt a gnawing on my insides for months about it and just didn't want to deal with it. Maybe he didn't either. People grow apart for whatever reason. It happens. It hurts, but it happens. And you can learn from the experience and heal. Right now, it is just incredibly painful. My devastation lies in now knowing some things that are making me question everything. Do you ever really KNOW someone? I thought I did, but now I don't know. I probably will never know and that is something I will just have to deal with. Everyone has issues, faults, character flaws, illnesses. You can't fix them for someone. You can't make them be what you think they should be or what you remember them to be. All you can do is be there, and we both did just that.

So my healing is really going to take awhile. Unfortunately, there is no timeline. Tough for the planner to know when she is going to be all healed up. The scars will fade, and my heart will heal. For more reasons than even I know, this is my new beginning.

What do you do when you start over? Do you make a bucket list? All the things you want to do, wish you could do? I guess I will figure that out with each passing day. I think rock climbing and sky diving will have to wait.

What I DO KNOW, is that I am strong. Stronger than I ever imagined myself to be. Strong enough to face my fears and deal with them head-on. I knew I would come out on the other side of this, but the process itself was nothing short of tormenting. Maybe "tormenting" is not the most accurate word. Taxing. That is the better word. Taxing to the point of mental, physical and emotional exhaustion.

But now I am done. Done with ALL of it. Done with surgeries (except for getting my new "girls"), done with chemo (HUGE) and done with a relationship with someone I truly loved, but didn't really know. There is no other way to put this than to say that it all SUCKS. But even things that suck find their way out of the blackness and get better.

I will find out this week the pathology of my thyroid biopsy. I am expecting all to be well, but will keep you all posted. For those of you who have e-mailed me to my home e-mail, I apologize. I have not been able to access those emails for a month. I know, RIDICULOUS. Another mess on my to-do-list to deal with.

Thank you all for continuing to call me, send me cards, and let me know that you are thinking of me. I think, all said and done, NOW is the time for cosmopolitans!

Love, Connie :)

Sunday, June 14, 2009 10:08 PM, CDT

Connie,

I am so glad to hear that you are almost done with it all. You are in the home stretch. I am so sorry to hear about you and Mark. (((hugs))).

SueAnn L.

Monday, June 15, 2009 8:39 AM, CDT

Connie, As I write this I do not know what words to type… "I'm sorry about Mark" seems so petty, while "I know you will get through this" seems so cold. You have been through so much and this is just one more thing added to your pile. You and only you can place this on the right pile. You will need to grieve, and hopefully not for long. If you ever need to talk, just call. I look forward to those cosmos!!!!!!!!!!!!!!

Love Judy G.

Monday, June 15, 2009 11:03 AM, CDT

Connie,

I am so sorry to hear about you and Mark. Time heals all wounds...You have been through so much, I can't even begin to imagine. You are a strong woman and I know you will get through all of this. Thinking about you and the kids and wishing you my best.

Debbie D.

Monday, June 15, 2009 3:59 PM, CDT

I know what you mean about questioning a lot of things. It is hard to think maybe there should have been some way to foresee it all, prevent it, change it, make it more bearable... take my advice and just let it all go...everything happens for a reason, including your marriage, divorce, meeting Mark, breaking up, even the "C" word. Only time will tell and heal all the wounds. So cliché, but would they be cliché if it wasn't how it usually goes down for just about everybody?? I love you Bramer. I know you are a strong beautiful woman and this is only the beginning of the rest of your story. Call me for the cosmos!! Love, Jen

Wednesday, June 17, 2009 7:11 PM, CDT

Each time I read your next chapter, Connie, I think "What more can happen?" And then, I find out. You have too many prayers being said for you to be walking alone through it all. I so wish this didn't have to happen to you, but it did, and you are stronger for going through it. A day will come when you will realize this was a time for more than just healing.

Love you, Connie and my prayers continue…Anna B.

Truth be told, I was beside myself. I lived through hell for what? To BE in hell when it was all over? Where is the fairness in that? My mother always said, "Life isn't fair." Well, NO SHIT Shirley! I feel so stupid. Like I've been had. The fool at her own party. So betrayed by lies, omissions, and illness. I found myself a tainted version of my old self. I knew more, had weathered more, but was I really wiser? Apparently not, as I sat there feeling foolish and alone. I was so angry and hurt.

Months of Mark not touching me, being my "pal" to watch movies with. I had spent all of that time wondering what was wrong with me. Was I repulsive somehow because I was sick? Because I was bald? How could he do this to me? All the time I spent feeling inadequate explained in a simple sentence: "I put my life on hold for you." Screw you! You HAD a life to put on hold. I was just hanging on to mine. I never asked him to put his life on hold for me. All I wanted was for him to be there for me because that's where I was hoping he wanted to be. Poor Mark, ever the hero, hanging in there with the girl who has cancer so he doesn't look like a jerk by walking away. Well, I would wash my hands of him, his lies, his mood swings and disappearing acts disguised as "bad sushi."

See ya.

So I embarked on my journey to wellness, wholeness and well, just plain fun.

Chapter 33
A New Beginning

Sunday, June 21, 2009 11:24 AM, CDT

Well, I'm done getting hacked up. No thyroid cancer!!! In all of this madness, I finally caught a break. Even my scars are looking a little less Freddy Krueger-ish. I've been putting so much vitamin E on my neck that if the light hit it just right, I probably could start a fire somewhere from the glare. So I WOULD be helpful on *Survivor*.

My hair is growing back. I seem to have the GI Jane look almost mastered. My friend Laurie came up to visit me yesterday (love you Laur—you're awesome!) and said I should go sans wig. Nah, I'm too self-conscious. Maybe in a few months. Wouldn't want to scare anyone unnecessarily.

My big news is that I am going to Ireland in less than 2 weeks! Me, on a whim. Imagine that! My dear friend Ellen and I are going. What a trip it is going to be! Ellen is no doubt my crazy twin in laughter. I can only imagine the laughs we are about to have, and boy, do I need them. I have never been to Europe and I just can't wait. All I can think about is the color green, as I am sure we will be seeing lots of it, pint after pint of Guinness beer and tons of laughter.

When I was in the middle of my chemo (sick as a freaking dog), I kept saying to myself, "I need to escape my life." Escape from cancer, escape from feeling like shit EVERY DAY. Escape from being tired, and in the midst of all of that having to be "on" as a mother. It was a lot to deal with at the time. So now I am going to have my week of escape to a beautiful countryside with an AMAZING friend for an experience of a lifetime. A week to heal from everything and somehow get myself back. My new adventures begin...

Warm wishes for all of my father friends and of course, my own wonderful dear old dad. Happy Father's Day!

Love,

Connie :)

My last journal entry. Sad to be done with the frequent verbiage of my escapades and adventures, but WOW, a new beginning. It is much the same as the feeling I had throwing my graduation cap in the air my last day of college. What next? I spent SO MUCH time being ill, do I even remember how to be well? And better yet, live well?

The road to recovery is slow. Meaning, it takes FOREVER for my hair to grow back. I'm so used to wearing my wig, it has become my security blanket. Much like the blanket Linus carries around with him in the *Peanuts* cartoons, but instead an added appendage of sorts. Each day that goes by, I examine my head for signs of improvement. I never thought losing my hair would be such a hardship. Aside from the many surgeries and chemo, it is my most reviled aspect of the cancer experience.

I plan a trip to Ireland, a spur of the moment decision that will result in the freeing of my spirit. My friend Ellen is the big sister I never had. The friend I look to for advice and wisdom, but most importantly the friend that I look at

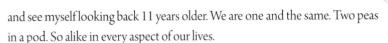

and see myself looking back 11 years older. We are one and the same. Two peas in a pod. So alike in every aspect of our lives.

The trip to Ireland is amazing. The countryside is breathtaking and every bit the patchwork quilt of green I always imagined. I saw this trip as my rebirth, a starting-over of sorts. A healthy me taking back my life.

It is an adventure of a lifetime, and at just the right time. I need to have fun, to forget about cancer. This trip is my start-over, my new beginning (sans hair of course), with the added joy of hot flashes that came on faster than the last one could dissipate. I had started on Tamoxifen which brought menopause with it like it was a free gift with purchase. Only this time, I had to go to the pharmacy for the prize, not the Lancôme counter.

I knew it would be a "trip" when Ellen's friend Bernie met me at the airport with a sign reading "Connie (Aer) Lingus." Don't ask. I flew Aer Lingus and my friend Ellen, of course, had to put her own spin on it.

We traipse around Ireland in a Yugo (yes, picture this), with Ellen's Irish friends captain and co-captain of the mother ship. Me in the backseat, taking in the sights, licking my wounds from Mark and thinking. Thinking about where I have just been and where I am going. We drive down into this valley of green and I sing, "The hills are alive, with the sound of music," to which Ellen adds, "aaahaha."

"Fecking Americans! You're crazy!" chimes a voice from the front seat.

Ireland is a place I will never forget, its shy beauty and kind people, like a soft light and lullabies with which to fall asleep at night. It is a peaceful place, and the perfect place for me to come to peace with my cancer and myself. I will be OK. I am on the road to getting myself back.

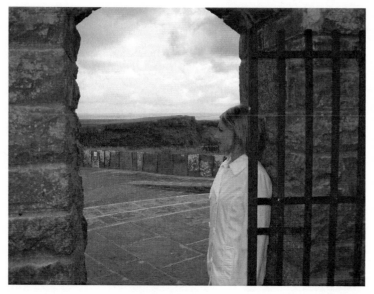

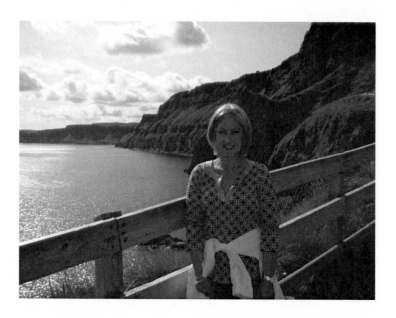

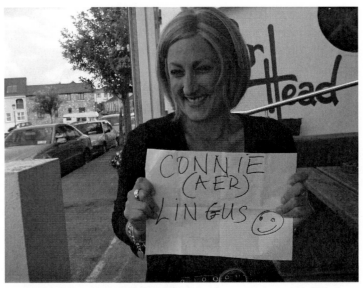

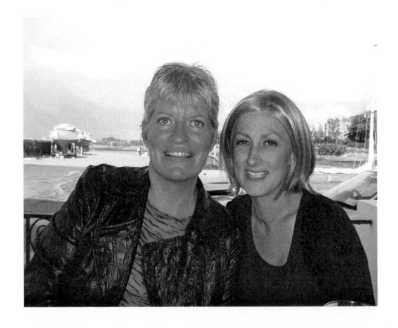

Later on that summer, I start to get my freak back. My chest expanders are filled with saline in preparation for my implants and I am feeling more comfortable in my clothes. Looking at me, no one would know I have been sick, except of course, for the wig. My brother comes up from North Carolina with his wife and we decide to head up to Saratoga for dinner. They come to pick me up, my brother and his wife, her sister and boyfriend. We pile in the car, head up to Saratoga and have to park in East Jesus because there is no parking as it is Saratoga in August and the town is in full swing.

We head downtown on foot. I'm feeling pretty good. The post-chemo coma seems to have subsided. I'm wearing a cute little sundress and heels. Let's face it, I'm looking pretty fabulous. As we walk down a side street, I duck under a tree branch and swoosh, my wig flies off my head, dangles in the branches of the tree and then slowly floats to the sidewalk below. It is as if I am watching it in slow motion.

I look around and everyone has their hands over their mouths, as if to say "Oh, shit!" I look at their faces and burst out laughing. There I am with maybe half an inch of hair on my head (that's being generous) and I bend over laughing so hard I can't breathe. THIS is by far the most hilarious situation I have ever been a party to and I'M the party!!!

My brother, who calls me "Cone," yells, "Cone, get the wig! Get the wig!" People walk all over both sides of the street. My posse looks mortified FOR me as opposed to AT me and I am still bent over laughing hysterically.

I bend down to get the wig, thinking "This must be quite the scene." Here I am bald, wearing a sundress and heels, bent down on the side of a busy street to retrieve my head squirrel. I wonder if there is a real squirrel in that tree secretly putting extra weight on the branch in order to capture the wig.

What a sight this is. I put the wig on my head, and it looks like the craziest mess of blonde, like the just-had-sex look. Except here, I am standing on the side of a busy street with people milling all around me. My brother yells to me, "Cone, calm that thing down!" So I stand, looking at my reflection in the window of a Jeep Cherokee, smoothing my wig down so as not to terrify the public passing by.

If Tom Bergeron had been around with a video camera, I would have for sure won the $100,000 prize. Damn, I could really use that money. I

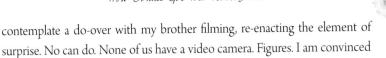

contemplate a do-over with my brother filming, re-enacting the element of surprise. No can do. None of us have a video camera. Figures. I am convinced my life is a real live comedy reel.

The following month, I hit another snafoo. Another infection with an expander, this time the left side. My surgeon removes the expander and by the grace of god, decides that I am well enough to have my implants put in that very same week. I'm all about having a nice rack, especially after all of the crap I have been through, so I opt for a C cup. The plastic surgeon measures this in cc's, not in handfuls, so a precise C cup is not possible. I have spent months being filled up to match my size of choice.

All of the breast surgeries are outpatient (thank god), and as I come awake from the anesthesia, I look down at my new chest and think, "Is this it?" They are much smaller than I remember my chest being just hours ago with the expanders. Definitely not a C cup! A C- at best. Well, at least I was still "passing." My doctor informs me there is a size differential between the expanders and the implants. Well, NO SHIT Sherlock! I had visions of myself much chestier and in this rocking hot pink bra I had picked out for my reveal.

Reveal to whom, I had no idea, but it's the visual I had in my mind after many months of scalpel encounters, chest drainage, and just plain annoyance. So now what? My surgeon informs me that I can go bigger, but he will need to order the implants and do this all over again. By this time, I am well over the five surgery mark, so my answer to that thought is HELL NO. I am SO OVER all of this. Maybe, I'll do it later...

Chapter 34
I Run For Life

*M*ight I just say that running and I are not friends. Acquaintances maybe. Playing soccer, I can run for a time as long as there is a ball somewhere in the vicinity that I am trying to conquer.

There were moments of pure restlessness during my months of treatment. Times where the only cure would be to throw on some sneakers and run, never looking back. Unfortunately, the energy level didn't quite match the mindset. I could envision the run, but then after a split second I'd say "Forget about it," traipse over to the couch with a bowl of ice cream and watch mindless television.

When I hit the midway point during my chemo, sporting my pink cotton hat, I announced to my nurses, "I am going to run the Susan G. Komen 5K in October." Shit, did I really just say that? Crap! Now I REALLY have to do it!

Honestly, the thought of making it through my chemo and running that 5K was all I had in my head. Even if I was sicker than a dog, I would do it. I had always supported the cause, but it was different now. It was MY cause. MY fight.

My cousin Don and his wife Patty were so generous as to sponsor shirts for my team to run the 5K. We had them made up to run in memory of my mother and in honor of myself and my friend Sue (from the Sue Crew). My friends Rene, Kim and Sharon walked with my kids. The run, well, that was my race.

My friend Cristina aka partner in crime and sorority sister, volunteered to run with me at my pace. I was very proud of myself as I ran almost the whole thing (had to walk a couple of times) with a not-too-shabby time if I do say so myself. It's funny to think that twenty years ago we were dancing on tables drinking beer and now, I was just so happy to be alive to run this race. The best feeling I had as I ran the race with my wig stuck on my head with a hat, was from the sound of cheers as I crossed the finish line.

I had always looked around at the "survivor" shirts in years past. Watched for signs of wear on the faces of so many women. To be truthful, every woman who wore that shirt, my new badge of honor, had a beautiful face full of hope and a spirit no one could squelch. I have learned that being a survivor bears not the perks of a club, but the extraordinary value of life and love. I felt a sense of relief at the finish line. I had made it.

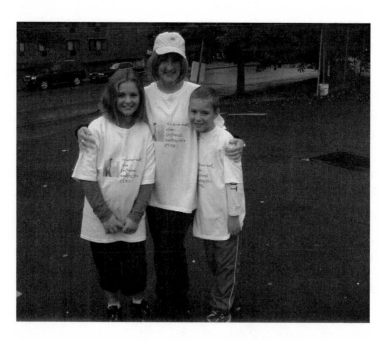

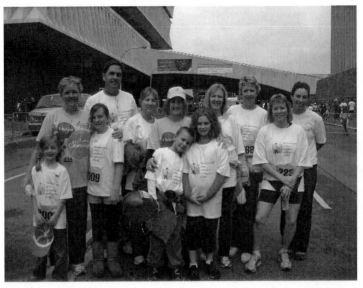

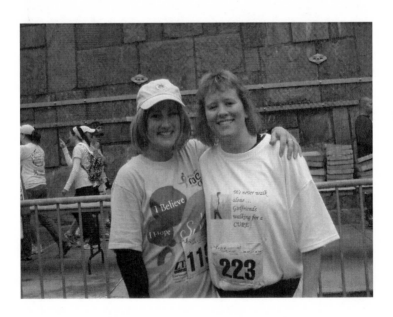

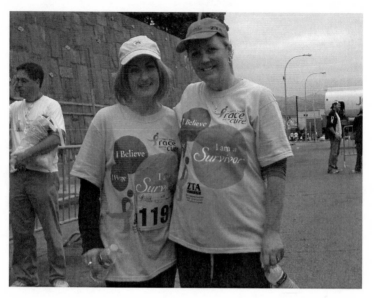

Chapter 35
Sisterhood

*T*here are many forms of sisterhood we encounter along life's journey. There are blood sisters, sisters by kinship of circumstance, and then there are sorority sisters. My sisters are bar-none some of the most exceptional women I know, and we did a lot of stupid shit together to become sisters in college.

I could foresee the demise of our on-campus reign during a Homecoming visit a few short years after graduating, when a current sister lifted her shirt at a keg party to reveal a double nipple piercing. Because of this, I think it is "safe" to tell this story. In order to explain the significance of a heartfelt gesture by my "sisters," I must disclose a pledge secret. Ladies, don't fret. I won't disclose everything, LOL.

Every Greek has to fulfill certain pledge tasks while pledging. One of our tasks was to hollow out an egg and have every sister sign it with purple ink. We carried our "IT" around in a yogurt container that we decorated and cushioned with cotton stuffing to keep it intact. The day before it was due, it was sitting in my backpack on the floor while I studied for a test at my desk. One signature short of completion, I got aggravated because I couldn't figure something out, slammed the book on the floor, on top of the backpack crushing the egg. HOLY SHIT! I just killed my "IT!" It took me TWO WEEKS to get those signatures! A fury ensued to create a new egg, gather more signatures and master my forging skills. For future pledge classes, I became known as the sister who killed my "IT."

A few months after my last chemo, I decide to go up to Homecoming weekend. It's funny because I almost bailed. I felt funny about going, especially since I was still wearing my wig.

I remember thinking, "Wow, there are a lot of sisters here." After going out to dinner, the ladies usher me into the hotel's great room and I saw a cake out of the corner of my eye. I was thinking maybe it was a birthday cake because my 40th birthday was later on in the month, but instead, they gathered around me and presented me with an oval-shaped box.

Inside the box was a porcelain ostrich egg with messages from my sisters written all over it in purple ink. They had shipped this egg back and forth across the country for months, writing me well wishes and messages of hope. I was speechless (which almost never happens). I could not believe that these women who I had partied with, sang songs with, and did silly things with, would go to so much trouble for ME!

I am so very grateful. This beautiful egg sits in its stand on my dresser. I look at it every day and read it often. It reminds me of where I have been, where I want to go and the love of truly amazing people. It is a gesture I will never in my life forget.

My sisters, my friends. Women of incredible integrity who have shown me that friendship IS for a lifetime. Thank you all from the bottom of my heart. (And yes, I wrote this completely sober!)

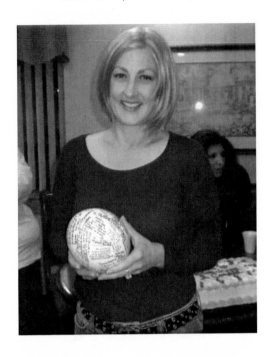

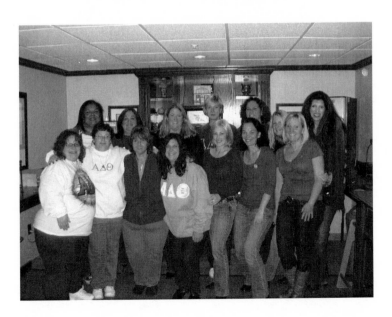

Chapter 36
Becoming Whole

After the implant surgery, I had several surgeries to correct the shapes of my breasts. When my surgeon told me that the hope for breast cancer reconstruction patients is that they can feel comfortable in a bathing suit and have cleavage for a low-cut top, I was completely crestfallen. "What about how I look naked? I look like I had a run-in with a bear in the woods and he smacked the shit out of my chest! Diagonal scars across both breasts, no nipples … must I go on?"

Apparently, my warped mind had me returning to a state of normalcy, nipples and all. Would I ever get to a point where I wouldn't think about cancer every time I looked in the mirror naked? The answer to that is, of course, no. But just like a horrible breakup can fade in pain, so can the memories of breast cancer. Every day that I am here beyond November 19, 2008 is a complete blessing.

I look forward to the time when my oncologist tells me that I don't need to see him again for a year. I can't adequately describe this, but once you have experienced chemotherapy, the smell of it evokes death like no other odor. As I enter the elevator on my way to his office, the smell hits me and I am back to a very bad place. A dark place with needles, medications I cannot pronounce, and an overwhelming feeling of dread that words cannot describe. Every three months I experience this, along with a fear of "Could it come back?" What if my bloodwork comes back and my cancer count is elevated?

My heart drops inside my chest at the thought. But I know, if cancer were to ever knock on my door again, I would stare it down and give it another run for its money. By now, I have had ten surgeries related to my cancer, including an oophorectomy (and no, it was not performed by oompa loompas as I first suspected). Suffice it to say, I think cancer is done with me. At least I hope so.

In my heart of hearts, I believe that my cancer journey has given me more than it has taken from me. So what? I don't have my own breasts anymore. I'm alive and now when I run, they stay in place. I have learned so much about myself. I know that I am stronger than I ever imagined, and that when faced with adversity, I have learned to compartmentalize. Now that I am through my journey, I can take cancer in its little box, put it on a shelf and forget about it.

I have learned that the love of your friends and family is what sustains you in hard times. My friends, and most importantly, my children, kept me from crawling into a dark place and staying there. My kids were amazing throughout my entire journey. Patient and wise, thoughtful and understanding. Quite remarkable for a seven and eight year old. And in turn, they have learned that no matter what life dishes out, you don't give up without a fight. I fought this fight for them, and they helped me to fight it for myself.

I want to thank everyone who has touched my life in some way or another. My dream team of doctors and nurses, family and friends. It is because of all of you that I am here. Alive and well, and sharing my story so that others may laugh and realize that a cancer diagnosis is not the end. It is a fork in the road that leads to a short detour of trials and tribulations, setbacks and triumphs.

Righting yourself and finding your way back to the main road is the challenge, but so worth the journey.

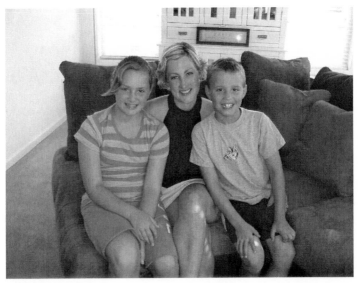

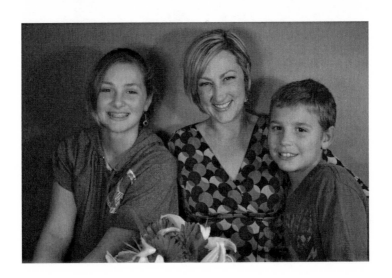

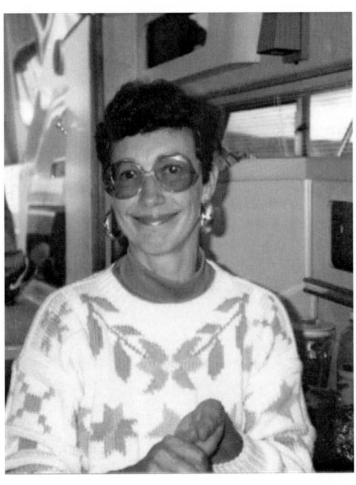

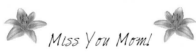 Miss You Mom!